HEALING

One of today's outstanding spiritual healers examines the origins of this ancient therapy and its application in Eastern and Western countries, and elaborates on the relationship between physical and non-physical problems and the central nervous system housed in the spine.

HEALING

The Energy that Can Restore Health

by

Bruce MacManaway
with Johanna Turcan

Series Editor

Dr George T. Lewith

THORSONS PUBLISHERS LIMITED
Wellingborough, Northamptonshire

First published March 1983
Second Impression July 1983
Third Impression 1984

British Library Cataloguing in Publication Data

MacManaway, Bruce
    Healing.
    1. Faith-cure
    I. Title   II. Turcan, Johanna
    615.8'52   RZ400

    ISBN 0-7225-0784-4
    ISBN 0-7225-0783-6 Pbk

Printed and bound in Great Britain

This book is dedicated to all those who through the millenia have endeavoured to enable humanity to discern, develop and apply their latent talents.

Bruce mac menaway

December 1984.

Acknowledgements

It would be impossible for me adequately to acknowledge all those who have influenced my thinking and understanding and therefore the content of this book.

My parents, Dick and Zelma, must head this list for their handling of my formative years. My mother and her twin sister, Iva Cosgrave, commenced their examination of the ESP faculties during the early 1930s, and thus were able to help me to rationalize the healing activity which expressed itself through me in 1940. I am happy to relate that they are still involved in helping others to discover and develop their abilities.

Inevitably, I risk causing offence by omitting mention of teachers and helpers who have contributed to my education. Some are anonymous or conceal their identities under pseudonyms—all invariably emphasize that we examine carefully the content of the communication rather than be influenced by the status of the communicator—'by their fruits shall ye know them'.

Many people, by and through whom my awareness has been expanded, include Louisa Ashdown, whose remarkable gifts I have never seen equalled, far less excelled, Grace Cooke, Harry Edwards, Sir George Trevelyan, Pir Vilyat Khan, Rimpoche Chogyam Trungpa, Father Andrew Glasewski and the Rev. Dr Kenneth Cumming. Through them, my attention was drawn beyond allopathic medicine into what is becoming known as complementary medicine, and similarly beyond Christian teachings towards those of other religions and philosophies.

Very importantly, I joyfully record the indispensible companionship of and help from my wife and sons who all have the gifts of healing and have shared whole-heartedly in building up the Westbank Centre.

Similarly, I am happy to share authorship with Johanna Turcan who, after a year in our home followed by several years of co-working, has shaped the material into readable form and prepared the bibliography. She and her parents have for many years supported and encouraged the development of the healing and teaching work and the centre from which we operate.

Lastly, I take this opportunity of thanking John Hardaker of Thorsons Publishers, and Dr George Lewith, the series editor, for entrusting me with this book and for painstakingly vetting the script and making valuable suggestions at each stage.

Contents

Foreword

Perhaps I should begin by declaring an interest. I believe in Bruce MacManaway's work because over the years I have had personal knowledge of it at different levels; and some of the experience he has had, I have had too. And I believe that he has something very important to contribute to the well-being of mankind.

First, the healing. Bruce discovered this gift in himself during the war when putting a hand on a wounded soldier to comfort him had the unforeseen effect of easing the soldier's pain. I came to realize something of what must have happened then the first time that Bruce put his hands on my back. Although I was wearing a shirt I felt as though a blow-lamp was being applied to my spine, the heat was so intense. Later, after interviewing for the BBC the late Harry Edwards (the man whom Bruce considers to have been this country's greatest healer), I asked if he could do anything to alleviate the congestion in my sinus. He put his fingers lightly on my cheekbones, and I felt the congestion melt away. I had no further trouble for two years.

Next, Bruce's dowsing techniques which he uses for analysis and diagnosis. When we met to discuss a television interview two remarkable things happened. The first was when my producer came and joined us. Bruce let his little dowsing pendulum run over his body: when it reached the general area of his hip, it began to oscillate. Bruce told the producer he had something wrong with his hip. The producer smiled, surprised; he had just had an operation on it.

Discussing this, Bruce said that the pendulum could also produce results from abstractions. When I asked what he meant, he said, 'Well, if you were to write down a list of simple questions on a piece of paper, ones that require a straight Yes or No, and turn the paper face downwards, the pendulum will come up with the correct answers.'

I was too sceptical of his claim to take it up with him then, but I made a mental note of it, and when the time came for the interview, I prepared a list of six questions (The Queen has ten children, Everest is the highest mountain in the world, etc) typed them on a piece of paper and put them in my pocket.

Half-way through the interview I brought out the piece of paper, reminded him of our previous conversation and asked if he would care to apply the pendulum to produce the answers. He said he would be delighted. So I put the questions on the table, face downwards, and he put the pendulum over them. He got the first one right, the second one right, the third one right, the fourth one right, the fifth one wrong and the sixth one right. What the odds were against this, I have no idea, but we were all enormously impressed. Bruce, though, was more concerned about the one that had got away, which he attributed to the artificial atmosphere created by the cameras and lights.

This is not all. In Chapter 9 Bruce describes a remarkable incident with a medium. I myself had a similar but less dramatic experience. Early in the war my father was killed while commanding H.M.S. Rawalpindi against two German warships. My mother subsequently attended several seances in which, she told me, he passed messages to her. Curious, I looked up the list of forthcoming seances advertised in my mother's copy of a Spiritualist magazine, and chose one at random.

Although in the navy myself, I went to the seance in civilian clothes. I was twenty-two and unknown publicly. The medium asked me to give her something personal and I gave her my ring, once my father's. She took it, then went into trance. 'I see the sea', she said, 'and a ship and the letter R and a battle. And there's someone connected with it who's very close to you.'

I have given these examples of extra-sensory experiences to show how greatly the scope of Bruce's work has expanded over the years, from the comparative simplicity of healing to embracing telepathy, dowsing, clairvoyance, levitation, ley lines, etc. Behind all this is his belief, based on the knowledge of man's age-old aspirations to union with a spiritual force, that we have neglected our intuitive sources of knowledge for too long. It is an awareness of and a reaching out for this, he believes, that can give us true health, make us integrated and whole. It is basically the same message that the world's religious leaders, philosophers and psychiatrists have always preached; that fragmented man is a sick man who can only be cured, as Plato said, by assessing mind, body and soul together.

Christ made no distinction between physical and spiritual well-being; for him they were indivisible and complementary. It was his followers in the mediaeval Church who set them apart, Bruce claims, to the lasting disadvantage of both. Who can doubt that he is right? If the Church had never become involved in the business of moral imperatives, never become authoritarian and censorious, concentrated instead on being a golden gateway to spiritual awareness, celebrated the living Christ rather than the dead one, what a different and more vibrant and altogether more helpful institution it might have been.

I feel as certain as Bruce does that if man is to find a way through the tangled thickets that lie ahead, he can only survive if he becomes more ready to respond to all the forces, visible and invisible, that shape him; if he listens rather less to the discordant voices of Presidents and Prime Ministers and rather more to what Keats called 'the spirit ditties of no tone'. It is less in the here and now and more in the intangible and unknowable that Bruce—and I—believe that man's best hope for the future lies.

LUDOVIC KENNEDY

Preface

I have tried to be as objective as possible in this book about healing. Many aspects that I touch on are now the subject of scientific research and are amply written up elsewhere. Healing is, however, a complex and at times emotive subject. Doctors, psychiatrists, nurses, numerous therapists, clergy, scientists and lay people of all sorts will approach it with their own concepts and beliefs. The subject can be rationally discussed within any chosen discipline, but trouble arises when, in attempting to extend our understanding of it, we use a shared concept but express it in terms that clash with someone else's beliefs. For example, such terms as spirit and soul may be acceptable to a cleric but they would be anathema to a scientist, and a psychiatrist may be happier with the terms psyche or subconscious.

It is inevitable, therefore, that at times some of my terminology will clash with your beliefs, particularly when my own rationale creeps in despite my stringent attempts to be objective. On these occasions I would ask you to refrain from choking on theory but to look at the underlying concept and see if it makes sense in different words. Better still, try the practice for yourself. There is no substitute for personal experience, and I know that I for one would have been but little impressed by the most learned treatise on healing when I first came across the phenomenon in 1940. I was convinced that healing worked only because I saw it do so with my own eyes and as a result of using my own hands under most inauspicious conditions.

I found that healing worked for me despite the fact that I knew nothing about it at the time. More than forty years later I still have no formal qualifications. I have been privileged to work with highly talented and skilled practitioners representing many varied medical, clerical and scientific disciplines. Inevitably I refer to work done or knowledge available, but I speak as a layman. If at times I oversimplify or misuse technical terms, please bear with me.

I hope that in the near future the various disciplines will be able to work more closely together. Over the last forty years I have seen tremendous changes, both in our scientific understanding of matters related to healing and in general attitudes. Even as I write, new discoveries are being made and the old barriers of intolerance are becoming less rigid. A great deal more remains to be done. More research needs to be carried out in the hospitals and clinics because, as yet, not nearly enough attention has been paid to proper 'follow up' studies of those patients who are receiving healing in addition to orthodox treatment. Attempts to help the sick take many forms of which medicine is perhaps the most important—healing should never be seen as a substitute for, far less a threat to, the medical world. We do need medical skills and knowledge more urgently than ever—but healing can assist the doctors in their task.

Introduction

Healing is often dismissed by the medical profession, but nevertheless it probably represents one of the most ancient systems of medicine. In this text, which I have had the privilege of editing, Bruce MacManaway has provided a clear and concise explanation of many of the ideas and beliefs involved in this field. His particular healing methods centre around the use of spinal and muscular manipulations, although he discusses many of the other methods involved in healing, such as 'the laying on of hands', 'absent healing' and 'dowsing'.

Since the Second World War a considerable body of scientific evidence has become available about healing, leading the enquiring reader to think very carefully before rejecting this therapy out of hand. While not claiming the case for healing is a proven one, it is important to assess the evidence in an objective manner. Bruce MacManaway has presented such facts as are available, but emphasizes the need for further research. He does not attempt to place healing on a pedestal as a somehow separate and mystical art, but encourages us to see how healing may work in conjunction with both conventional and alternative therapies.

All medicine and medical men have a little of the healer in them. Conventional therapy may call this a placebo response, but whatever terms are used, people can make other people well without using a specific therapy. It would be wise for us all to consider this before becoming too over-enthusiastic about a particular treatment.

GEORGE LEWITH M.A., M.R.C.G.P., M.R.C.P.,
Southampton, 1983

1. Concept and Historical Background

The concept of healing by touch or thought without any medical help does not fit comfortably into our Western view of the world. Yet we still retain some vestiges of it in everyday life. If a child has a temperature, we know that sometimes we can calm him by smoothing his brow. When calm, his fever may diminish and he will be able to sleep, giving his body rest and the opportunity to combat illness.

What is this, after all, but the interaction between two people, a communication between caring adult and child or between healer and patient? Outside the family context, we all know of people who respond to one medical practitioner, having shown no improvement when treated by another with identical qualifications and even using the same treatment. 'Bedside manner', we call it; 'something to do with giving the patient psychological or emotional confidence', we may add.

But what is that 'something'? Is it some psychological approach on the part of the practitioner? Does it point to some psychological factor in the patient which needs attention before recovery can commence? Nobody knows exactly. But to the extent that it is possible to add an extra 'something', a multitude of those in the caring professions, be they doctors or nurses or any one of the many skilled therapists, are already practising healing. They are in fact using a gift as well as their knowledge, skill and patience and are opening themselves to respond to the patient's unspoken needs. This factor, which is currently played down, should surely be developed and used to the utmost of our capacity. We do not attach any but the vaguest labels to it at the moment and it deserves very serious consideration.

The Concept of Healing
I should say that the communication between healer and patient sets up an interplay of energy which accelerates the patient's own internal healing processes. This, amongst other things, enables him to respond more fully to orthodox treatment. From this it should be seen that

while healing can and does achieve some astonishing results, it is not competing with orthodox medicine, nor seeking to supplant it. Surely it makes sense to use everything possible in the fight to restore and maintain individual health, and the many approaches should be complementary. I hope that healing will become one of the next in the long line of initially unacceptable practices which have subsequently been acknowledged and incorporated into orthodox medical practice. The list includes antiseptics, anaesthetics, orthopaedics and psychology.

Background

Before scientific medicine developed, healing in some form played a much larger role. Herbalism and other nature cures were important, but the power of healing on its own without recourse to other therapy has been known for thousands of years, and is still taken for granted in some societies (or the remnants of them) today. In the U.S.A. in 1981 I met a number of North American Indians and was introduced to some of their wise men! None of them was at all surprised by my work.

The Tibetans who have left their homeland have brought with them enormous esoteric knowledge, including a great understanding of healing. One of their Supreme Abbots visited us in Scotland. I was earnestly trying to describe to him what we try to do in our Centre, but he cut me short with a gentle smile. 'We would regard what you are doing as orthodox medicine. Amongst Tibetans, it is your Western doctors who are regarded as unorthodox.' Explanations were unnecessary and we realized that he, of course, knew a great deal more about the subject than anyone in the West.

Healing was known to the Chinese as far back as 5000 B.C. and subsequently in virtually every culture. In Egypt, all cures were originally thought to be revealed by the gods and codified by Thoth, known to the Greeks as Hermes Trismegistus. They were recorded in secret books for initiates kept in the medical schools associated with the temples of Sais at Heliopolis.

It seems that the earliest figure known for his healing powers is a man called Imhotep. He was court architect and court magician to King Zoser of the third Egyptian dynasty who lived about 2,700 B.C. After his death he was deified and his tomb seems to have become the Lourdes of the ancient world. Numerous temples and shrines were erected to him and the sick were brought to them for healing. Imhotep was thought to inhabit the body of a snake, a symbol which has since recurred frequently in relation to healing, not least in the winged staff and serpent of the Western medical profession today.

The Edwin Smith Surgical Papyrus indicates that the Egyptians had considerable rational knowledge of medicine, but this was not divorced from religion, and various gods and goddesses such as Seklimet and Amenophis were considered to play an important part in sickness and cure. The cult of Imhotep seems to have been the most famous, however, as it spread via Persia to ancient Greece where the god was called Asklepios. The remains of healing temples and shrines dedicated to Asklepios can still be seen on the island of Epidaneos. The cult then spread to Rome in the third century B.C. where the god became known as Aesculapius.

Healing in the past was usually inextricably tied with religion, but then so was virtually every other aspect of life. All knowledge and learning was based in the temples, and the gods were considered to permeate and influence all the workings of man and his environment: the harvests, the rainfall, peace and war, sickness and health. All education, both what we would regard as secular as well as religious, was only available through the temples, and the wisdom acquired by the priests and priestesses and wise men and women (known in Egypt as the Scribes of the House of Life),[2] was of a high order, even if it was not recognized as independent of supernatural forces.

The wisdom and the power might be learned within the inner circle of a particular cult, but in many societies the initiates could then demonstrate very considerable powers to the rest of the population. Well known examples would include the yogis in India, the medicine man of North America and the Shamans in parts of Africa, Asia and elsewhere.

Religion and Science
It was the Greeks who laid the foundations of Western thought. From the concept of an integrated universe in which man, matter, mind and life forces, often identified as gods, were inextricably linked, a mechanistic, analytic viewpoint ultimately emerged which divided the world as man perceived it in separate unrelated compartments.

This led to the beginning of a scientific approach to medicine in the context of the belief that while the supernatural might perhaps interfere, the universe ran on mechanistic lines which man could ultimately master.

Western thought has developed from this point and it became axiomatic to despise most of the knowledge of the ancient cultures (or indeed the latter 'backward' societies) because of their underlying unscientific approach. It is worth commenting in passing that Western dependence on logic and science has led to a certain intellectual blindness. It has been able to dismiss all the old knowledge because of the 'superstitious' way in which it was expressed. Because Western thought could not appreciate the theory, it assumed the practice was beneath its notice. But the practice of engineering, for example, as shown by the cities of the Incas or the building of the pyramids should have given us a clue to the fact that however 'primitive' the beliefs, the knowledge, in practice, was exceedingly impressive. If, selectively, we have to accept some of the knowledge because of the remaining concrete proof, can we uncompromisingly dismiss the rest?

Over the last two thousand years the Western approach to medicine and healing has been moulded by two factors. One is the slow but accelerating development of science. The other is religion. Whatever the current state of religious belief, the Western world is firmly founded on the profound influence of Christianity or perhaps more accurately, on the influence of the Church. The two have not always been easy bedfellows and have at times led to double intellectual standards. I came across this for the first time in 1943. I had no intention of becoming a healer but having discovered while fighting in France three years earlier that I seemed to be able to help my wounded companions, I had no good reason to withhold any help I could give thereafter. During the North African Campaign, however, I ran into an officer who regarded my spare time activities with horror. I was used to friendly, tolerant disbelief and the argument that every intelligent, educated man must know perfectly well that what it was claimed I could do was nonsense. It was unscientific. It was impossible. But this was the first time I met the reaction that if lay healing was possible, then it shouldn't be allowed. A cleric who had bravely given up his cloth to join the army, this particular officer was convinced that only an ordained priest could invoke the power of God for healing. Anyone else, if they were not charlatans or deluded, must be in league with the Devil. I have our regimental chaplain to thank for getting me out of what promised to be a full scale row. He had known my grandfather who was Bishop of Clogher and apparently persuaded my superiors that MacManaways were strange but harmless.

The 'doublethink' that lay healing can't happen but if it does, it shouldn't, has a long history.

Teachings of Jesus and the Early Church

Jesus of Nazareth was born in a country where, and at a time when, a number of cultural influences intermingled. Egyptian, Greek, Roman, Persian and even Indian ideas were all in evidence and healers were not unknown. It is not denying His Divinity to say that He was a superb, perhaps unique exponent of the gift or power of healing, but He did not present something intrinsically new.

Some of the Dead Sea Scrolls indicate that healing not unlike that practised by Jesus was being taught before He was born. The sect who left us the Dead Sea Scrolls may have been Essenes who, according to the Roman historian Flavius Josephus (first century A.D.), undoubtedly practised various forms of healing.[3] Some authorities in fact argue that Mary and Joseph were Essenes and that Jesus received his early education in the temples of the Therapeutae, the Egyptian counterparts of the Essenes, in the years after fleeing from Herod.[4]

Jesus is emphasized as not only the Son of God but also the Son of Man. He instructed His followers (and here let us remember that He was not addressing scholars or doctors or priests but ordinary men and women) to go and put into practice what He had shown them. He emphasized that His followers had the potential to achieve even greater things than He, so presumably considered that man could, amongst other things, heal (St John 14:12). As a great spiritual teacher, He also emphasized that man must use this potential with care and follow His spiritual path.

St Luke, of course, could hardly be described as a layman as he is thought to have been a qualified physician. Tradition has it that he was also a healer, probably trained at a temple of Asklepios in Greece. He therefore represents to me the best of both worlds, having a developed gift of healing *and* medical training. I count myself extremely lucky to have known and worked with a number of gifted doctors who are overtly reviving this tradition of combining healing and medicine and I greatly hope that it will spread once more.

During the first and second centuries, the early Church endeavoured to carry out Jesus' teaching. There is considerable academic argument as to whether the early Church was ever purely a gathering of exponents of the Spirit or whether it had in it from the start the makings of an organization.[5] It is beyond doubt, however, that at least during the lives of the Apostles what we would now call the charismatic gifts (healing, the gift of prophecy and speaking with tongues being the most obvious) were practised by men, and in many cases women, at the early services. These services were informal, held in private households and bore more of a resemblance to a Quaker meeting where anyone is free to express himself as the Spirit moves him (or her) than to a modern church service.[6] The Church in Corinth which was under the influence of St Paul was particularly famed for this and indeed St Paul wrote a wonderful essay on these gifts (the 'gifts of the Spirit') in his first letter to the Corinthians, chapters twelve to fourteen.

Broadly speaking, however, it would seem that from the earliest stages, there were two groups who might have some claim to authority over the Church members. One group included the healers and prophets who by their gifts demonstrated their contact with the Spirit. The other group was officialdom, the bishops and priests. That the priests found their authority threatened by the healers and prophets is obvious from the various documents in which the Christians were exhorted to show respect and duty to the Bishops. *The Didache,*[7] which probably dates from the middle of the second century, admonishes its readers: 'Therefore despise (the bishops and deacons) not, for these are they which are honoured of you with the prophets and healers.' Surrounded as they were by internal and external threats (persecution, schism and alternative cults such as neo-Platonism, Manicheism and the Mystery Cults), the early Church authorities were in something of a quandary. They did not wish to stop the activities of the healers (or at least they did not wish to be seen to be doing so) but they wanted unity and order. The crunch came over a group of churches in Phrygia in Asia Minor where Montanus and his followers, and in particular two very gifted women, were gaining a dangerous amount of influence by their prophesying and healing. According to the historian Tertullian, a priest called Praxeus[8] was largely responsible for persuading the Bishop of Rome to excommunicate the affected churches and brand their members as heretics.

From the point of view of lay healers, this decision was, to say the least, discouraging. They could either keep quiet and stay within the organization of the faith they passionately believed in, or continue their practises and risk being thrown out in the cold. Ultimately, there was an effective if unspoken ban on lay healers. The ordained priests, while usually good and holy men, were more concerned with theology and with administration than healing.

With Constantine's conversion and the gradual adoption of Christianity as the predominant state religion, what had previously been a Church ban acquired all the penalties of secular law and for a layman to practise any of the gifts of the Spirit became a very risky business. The practising of the gifts within the auspices of the Church was allowed and the Church has had its 'saints'. Even they, however, were and are grilled pretty thoroughly before gaining acceptance. Anyone outside the Church's control ran the risk of the accusation of heresy or witchcraft with the concomitant danger of death. Until as late as 1951, I and others like me ran the theoretical risk of arrest under the Witchcraft Act which carried the death penalty, even if it had not been used for some time. By claiming a monopoly of the gifts of the Spirit, the Church has alternately brainwashed and bullied the population into thinking that any person trying to heal without the proper qualifications must be in league with the Devil. I maintain that this is not in accordance with the teachings of Christ himself, who lived and taught amongst laymen. It is not surprising, however, that healing went underground.

The Age of 'Enlightenment'

Leaving aside the religious connotations for the moment and regarding healing as an observed phenomenon practised in other civilizations before and after Christ, its suppression was completed by the tremendous intellectual progress of the West, culminating in the view that anything inexplicable by intellectual means could not exist. Luckily, a little of the knowledge was maintained underground. Rather like the bumble-bee which continues to fly despite the fact that its flight is considered to be aerodynamically impossible, those unimpressed by current logical conclusions continued to practise what, to their satisfaction, demonstrably worked.

Current Intellectual Attitudes

In the light of recent progress, there is a need to reassess our understanding of the universe and our relationship with it. Our contempt for the ancient—and in fact still current—esoteric knowledge was that it was at best mystical and at worst superstitious and as such was unscientific and bore no relationship to reality. 'Reality' was based on an objective, scientific analysis of matter. Matter was solid, matter was concrete, matter was made up of 'building blocks' subject to comprehensible laws of cause and effect. Mind was totally separate and could have no 'real' effect on the mechanics of matter. In the context of human health, demonstrable disease was purely a mechanistic problem. The matter which makes up the human body was decaying or malfunctioning and the only way to combat this was to tinker with the mechanism, adding something here or subtracting something there. But, apparently, matter is not nearly so uncomplicated as we thought it was. According to modern physicists, it is not concrete at all, as even the atom is not a satisfactory 'basic building block'. Apparently, especially in 'quantum-relativistic' models of the subatomic world, totally objective study is impossible as any experiment inevitably includes the observer in an essential way[9].

I am no scientist, but it would seem to me that this means we can no longer regard 'matter' (which includes our own bodies) as something 'outside' and objective, divorced from mind. Perhaps disease is not such a simple mechanistic problem after all. Perhaps, at least in concept, the idea of healing is not totally outrageous. Perhaps the old (and current Eastern) concepts of a dynamic, inseparable universe were not far from the truth, even though they had no scientific basis.

In this new, humbler spirit of enquiry, some scientists have started to look around for some observed phenomena that they can measure which might be related to and cast light on the preposterous but tenacious claims for healing. Healing, as it needs no 'matter' to be supposedly efficacious, seems to depend on mind, so the obvious place to start was with the electrical patterns of the brain. It has been discovered that certain distinctive and unusual brain wave patterns are found in most supposedly effective healers, regardless of what they believe.

In the past, abilities such as healing had been associated with some form of religious or spiritual training, so the researchers studied some Eastern Holy men as well as healers in the West. They found that the various Holy men showed patterns similar to those of the healers, though in many cases the patterns were of even greater strength[10]. This research merits more discussion but for the moment it seems to me that it highlights two points. If people with a wide variety of beliefs or with no belief at all and united only in their purported abilities show a similar unusual brain wave pattern, it is probable that it is state of mind rather than belief that is important—though it may be that a strong religious belief is one of the variables affecting states of mind.

Secondly, religion and science may not be quite so far apart after all —or at least a bridge may be formed between the two if it can be shown that various religions and spiritual disciplines achieve special measurable states of mind that in turn can be associated with physiological changes. 'Religion', in its widest sense, may have known a thing or two, even if it was wrapped up in mystical language.

I will refer to further scientific research later but, while it is comforting that some scientific rationale is being built up, it is not my only concern. This book merely attempts to put forward some facts and some theories about what works, and as science is confirming, does so regardless of belief.

To state outright at this point that healing is natural rather than supernatural and works regardless of belief is likely to offend those who think of it as a God-given gift. I would say that the two attitudes are not mutually exclusive. Firstly, the fact that healing was known and practised before the birth of Jesus and later in ignorance of His teaching, gives more rather than less validity to Jesus' message. There is after all considerable point to Kipling's question, 'What should they know of England who *only* England know?'

Secondly, just because we find some rationale behind an observed phenomenon is not to say that the phenomenon is not God-given. Playing the violin, for example, is considered a natural talent, though undoubtedly some people play it better than others. The gift for playing the violin may come from God, but it is not a supernatural activity. The virtuoso may or may not believe in God, but he plays superbly anyway, and God does not appear to be small-minded enough to take away his ability to transport listeners to the heights because His part has not been given full credit.

So while the spiritual, God-given aspect of the healing gift is to me very important, healing can nevertheless be viewed on its own as a natural phenomenon.

Bibliography
1. See, for example, Storm, Hyemeyohsts. *Seven Arrows*. Ballantine Books U.S.A., 1972.
2. Sauneron, Serge. *The Priests of Ancient Egypt*. Evergreen Books, London; Grove Press, New York.
3. Allegro, John. *The Dead Sea Scrolls, a Reappraisal*. Penguin Books, 1964.
4. Hiebel, Frederick. *Treasures of Biblical Research and the*

Conscience of the Times. Anthroposophical Press, 1970.

Steiner, Rudolf. *Fifth Gospel*. Rudolf Steiner Press, 1968.

——. *Gospel of Matthew*.

——. *Christinaity as Mystical Fact*.

Cayce, Edgar. *Early Christian Epoch, Vol. 6*.

Szekely, Edmund Bordeaux. *The Discovery of the Essene Gospel of Peace*.

——. *The Essene Jesus*.

——. *The Gospel of the Essenes*.

5. Wand, J. W. C. *A History of the Early Church to A.D. 500*. Methuen, 1975; University Paperback, 1977.

6. Tertullian. 'On the Soul' ('De Anima'), quoted in *A New Eusebius, Documents Illustrative of the History of the Church to A.D. 337*. SPCK, 1957. (It is disputed whether this document describes a Catholic or Montanist service.)

7. Quoted in *A New Eusebius*.

8. Tertullian. 'Against Praxeus' ('Adversus Praxean'), quoted in *A New Eusebius*.

9. Capra, Frithjof. *The Tao of Physics*. Fontana, 1976.
For a thoroughly readable summary of what he calls 'the perversity of physics' see also: Koestler, Arthur. *The Roots of Coincidence*. Pan Books, 1976.

10. Cade, C. Maxwell and Coxhead, Nona. *The Awakened Mind*. Wildwood House, London, 1980.

2. Current Attitudes and Research

Despite that fact that science is forcing us to re-examine the old views of what is possible and what is impossible, the traditional authorities on healing, namely the medical establishment and the Church, understandably regard any claimants on their preserves with caution and suspicion. This is not true of individuals within these institutions and I have been privileged to work with many doctors and clergy of all denominations over the years and have been immensely grateful for their co-operation and help.

The hierarchy of the Church of Rome has been especially sympathetic towards healing in my experience. I first came under the Vatican's eye in 1946 when I was stationed in Rome and spending a great deal of my spare time working not only with my fellow British but with many Italian families I met. The Jesuit who investigated my activities took the matter up with his superiors. I was thrilled beyond measure to be told ultimately that I might inform any Roman Catholics who had doubts about coming to me for healing that they could write for authority to the Vatican, as Pope Pius XII had taken a personal interest.

I was delighted and grateful to find similar encouragement when I was again in Italy in 1957, attached to an Italian regiment. Once again my healing activities had brought me to the attention of the Catholic authorities. One thing led to another and finally I was privileged to meet the then Archbishop of Venice, later to become Pope John XXIII. He too told me that any Catholics in his diocese who were worried might write to him for authority to come to me for healing.

I found the same tolerant, understanding attitude in this country when the late Monseigneur Ronald Knox signified to a Roman Catholic priest of my acquaintance that he would give similar authority to any Catholic who wrote to him.

Unfortunately, neither the medical nor the religious authorities in this country have carried out any official research into lay healing on a significant scale in recent years. It is perhaps a little unfair to bring up reports that were produced nearly thirty years ago but as they are still frequently quoted, I would like to give my side of the story.

It was in 1953 that the Archbishops of Canterbury and York set up a Commission on Divine Healing (they later dropped the word 'Divine') with the help of some specially appointed doctors. I was involved with this and with a similar BMA commission and found both of them equally frustrating. The doctors appointed to carry out the research by the BMA started by asking the various healers they were supposed to investigate to produce the medical records of any patient they wished to put forward as an example of successful healing. I do not know if you have ever tried to obtain possession of your own medical records, far less those of anyone else. They are the closely guarded property of the patient's medical advisers, and a healer does not officially come into this category. Those of us who had been asked to participate and had willingly put ourselves forward for examination promptly pointed out that we would be unable to produce the official records for reasons well known to our examiners. We suggested that, instead, the examining doctors should themselves carry out some studies of patients before and after treatment and liaise on an official professional basis with the patients' doctors. Our suggestion was not taken up and we were told that if we could not produce medical records, further research was impossible. Similary, the Church Commission apparently did not follow up any of the cases put forward by the healers, or check the records which they (but not the healers) could so easily have done.

Not a single reference to the evidence for healing (good or bad!) which had been made available to the Church Commission appeared in their report, as apparently such an enquiry had not come within the Commissioners' terms of reference. *Can* one prepare a report without looking at or referring to the evidence? It is hardly surprising that the report said that 'No actual authenticated case of extraordinary and medically impossible healing has been brought to the Commission's notice.' They did admit that 'if the investigation was sufficiently complete there might arise scientific evidence for unparalleled physical cures' and they were 'not prepared to say that no such healings had ever occurred.'

The two commissions concluded that any cure or partial cure that is claimed to have resulted from healing is in fact due to wrong diagnosis, wrong prognosis, suggestion, remission or spontaneous healing. The two latter explanations are surely only ways of saying that something has happened but no one knows why.

Remission and spontaneous healing are well known and if they occur *after* the patient has received healing, this is no proof that they occurred *because* of the healing treatment. It is most unfortunate, however, that these commissions did not look more carefully at the evidence to see if, by any chance, spontaneous recovery happened more frequently after healing than coincidence would allow.

Suggestion and the Placebo Effect

Airily to dismiss any medically inexplicable cure or healing as the result of suggestion is surely unfair. Medicine is already well aware of the fact that belief or 'suggestion' can make people better. If someone believes that pills from the doctor will cure their symptoms, then time and again pills from the doctor will do so—even if the pills contain nothing more potent than sugar and colouring. But why does this happen? We recognize this so-called 'placebo effect', but we underrate it. Surely the vital point is that health is restored and the fact that we do not fully understand what triggers off the individual's own healing processes is bad for our intellectual egos but of secondary importance. If it works, then the patient is happy even if the physician is puzzled, so long live the placebo.

It is highly probable that healing sometimes works on the placebo principle. Undoubtedly, one is off to a head start if the patients themselves believe they are going to get better, whatever the basis of their belief may be. Some may already be sincerely religious and feel that God can heal them through someone else. Many come for healing because they have found themselves on the medical scrap-heap and make themselves believe in healing as a desperate last resort. The placebo effect undoubtedly cannot be ruled out of healing, *just as it cannot be ruled out of orthodox medicine*. I say again, if people get well, God bless the placebo.

This is not the whole story, however. Experiments with encephalographs which I will describe later in this chapter indicate that healing can bring about changes in the patient regardless of the patient's attitude, short of aggressive non-co-operation. In addition, I have frequently been surprised by the speed with which small pre-language children and animals will respond to healing. They obviously cannot believe in anything, although the child can respond to feelings from the mother and the animal to its owner, and I suspect that if the mother or owner felt reassured this could be transmitted to the patient.

Healing Guilds and Services

I am not at all sure where the Church of England now stands officially in its attitude to lay healing. The Churches Council for Health and Healing is doing valuable work. It is also exciting to see so many healing guilds springing up within the churches of all denominations and to hear of the dedication and success of healing services.

The General Medical Council

The doctors' professional association, the BMA, still takes a fairly

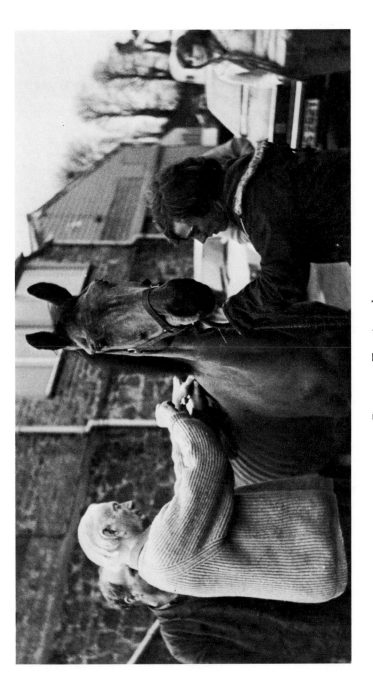

Figure 1.   Treating a horse.

hostile approach to healing. In their 1980 handbook it is flatly stated that doctors should not refer patients to osteopaths and by implication to any other practitioners of 'alternative' medicine. On the other hand, the General Medical Council, which is established by law to oversee the medical profession, takes a more tolerant view and does not restrict connections with 'alternative' practitioners! This position was reiterated in the recent report of the Royal Commission on the National Health Service.

In June 1981, I myself received a letter from the General Medical Council. It referred to the Council's Guidelines on Professional Conduct and Discipline in relation to the delegation of treatment to nurses or other persons who have been trained to perform specialized functions. While it is clear that the Council does not consider healers to fall into this category, the letter states that it is 'open to a doctor to suggest or agree to one of his patients seeking assistance from another source which he feels might be of benefit to the patient provided that the doctor himself continues to give, and to remain responsible for, any medical treatment he considers necessary for the patient and is able to ensure that there is no interference with the treatment which he may have prescribed in the case.' I have never regarded healing as in opposition to medicine but as a useful supplement. I am therefore delighted that at least it is now officially permissible for doctors and healers to work together.

I can understand the authorities' reluctance to give blanket acceptance to lay healers as there is not enough official verification of their effectiveness. Such a statement rather begs the question of why more official research has not been carried out. More and more healers are appearing in this country. One would have thought that no one would go to a healer except as a last resort and the fact that increasingly large numbers of people are doing so surely raises a number of points. Is the population becoming more gullible? Is the medical profession so overworked that people go elsewhere? Does healing really help large numbers of people? I must make a strong plea that more official research is badly needed, including extensive 'before and after studies' of patients who have received healing.

Varieties of Healing

One of the difficulties from the point of view of anyone trying to assess healing is the lack of consensus on theory. There are almost as many variations in and theories about healing as there are practitioners. While numerous healers will agree on certain points, they may each have their pet theories and their own specialities. Perhaps the most important factor that is recognized by most (but not all) of the healers I have met is the existence of some force or some energy outside themselves that they can channel but for which they are not responsible.

If the healer is only a channel, he cannot claim for himself the credit for any cures or assistance he may give. Opinion varies about this force that is channelled, so that healing has been given many names, spiritual healing, faith healing and magnetic healing being the best known. In the case of magnetic healing, the theorists would not claim any form of consciousness behind the force they use, but they may nevertheless recognize some external factor which they can feel and use. Recognition of some external force is not essential, however. Many healers do not think they are 'channels' and are nevertheless very effective. Once again, while my own beliefs are important to me, I prefer to leave them out of my definition of healing because I cannot stress too strongly the fact that healing *works*, regardless of belief. For this reason, I prefer to stick to the plain term 'healing' without any descriptive prefixes.

Many healers use therapeutic aids to supplement their healing gift or concentrate on one particular part of the body as the key to the general health of the patient. Therapeutic aids range from colour and light to herbal remedies and gems. Any or all of these may have 'objective' therapeutic powers, scientifically proven or otherwise. Parts of the body that receive attention include the eyes (iridology) and the feet (reflexology). I myself pay particular attention to the spine and, like anyone with a pet theory, I will go to great lengths to insist that the spine, or more properly the nervous system housed within it, is vital and the most important factor of all.

I suspect that what matters in all of these methods is the individual's capacity as a healer as much as the aids or therapies that he uses. Any or all may indeed have objective validity, (and I shall certainly claim objective importance for the spine), but I still maintain that the practitioner is more important than the practice. I have seen Harry Edwards correct spines, free siezed-up joints and alleviate all manner of conditions by no more than putting his hands on a patient.

'Simple' Healing and the Laying on of Hands

Healing, at its simplest, is merely a reaction between two or more persons. You may well say that this is not anything very new or original. We all know people whose mere presence cheers us up (or the reverse!); it may be their sheer exuberance, their personality, or some other factor which we do not bother to define. The reaction they can induce is neither as vague nor as undramatic as it sounds. Current slang provides a pointer. One hears the expression 'good vibes', or we talk of finding ourselves 'in tune' with someone. This is symbolic language, representing a reality which is not yet fully understood.

Our sense of touch is enormously important to us in establishing our understanding of the world around us. It is also a means of communicating. While it is perfectly possible for a reaction between two people to happen, regardless of physical proximity, touch does help. The laying on of hands is probably the oldest and simplest form of healing. We still retain vestiges of it in its simplest form in that, if a child is feverish, it is instinctive to smooth his brow. Sometimes, this is all that is required to calm the child. If not, we call the doctor. Between the mere stroking of a child's brow and the miracles of Jesus, there is a great gulf, but they are both, I think, extreme examples of some healing capacity in man.

Unfortunately for the rest of us, there are very few healers in any age who approach Jesus' abilities. This is not to say that supposed miracles are gone forever; Jesus was, after all, the Son of Man, and He did emphasize that we should go and do greater things than He. For most of us, however, a middle way must be sufficient, and while the laying on of hands can do a very great deal, we need to make use of the therapies and the vast medical knowledge as well.

'Tuning In' to Other People and Biofeedback Discoveries

What actually happens when a healer places his hands on a patient? Some research work into healing involves the use of encephalographs, machines which monitor the rhythms of electrical activity originating in the brain? I have been privileged to work in the last five years with Maxwell Cade, one of the foremost researchers in this field. As a fellow of the Institute of Electrical Engineers, a member of the Institute of Physics, a member of the Institute of Biology, a fellow of the Royal Society of Medicine and an Honorary Member of the National Council of Psychotherapists, he is peculiarly well qualified to co-ordinate the many highly technical skills required for such research. He has tested numerous healers in this country and has found that they produce a very unusual brain wave pattern when they are working with a patient. More surprisingly, they impose the same pattern on the patient, a pattern that the patient cannot produce on his own without special training. This conclusively demonstrates the reality of healer and patient 'tuning in'.

While it is of interest to discover that healer and patient do get on to the same wave-length, so to speak, it does not get us very far unless the particular pattern can be associated with beneficial physiological results. Maxwell Cade, Dr Ann Woolley Hart and many others have for some time been exploring the possibilities of measuring sensitive physical and mental reactions and have developed a variety of machines which give an immediate reading. Work in this field goes under the general term of biofeedback and the basic principle is very simple: if one is physically enabled to observe some biological happening in oneself, of which one is not normally aware, then one can be trained to control that happening. This has enormous implications for self-help, (in reducing one's own blood pressure without drugs, for

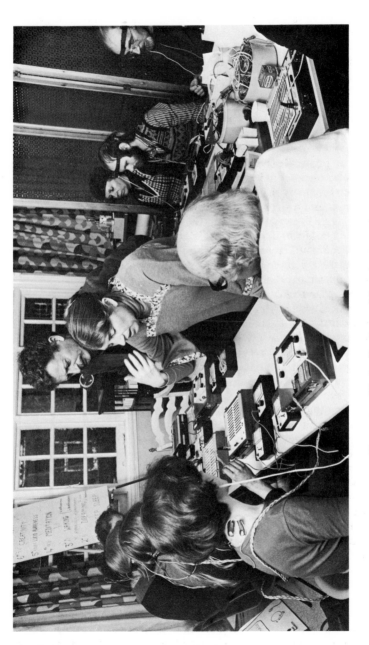

Figure 2. Biofeedback machines in operation.

example), but from the point of view of research into healing, it means that a feeling of healing can be seen on these sensitive machines to have a physiologically measurable correlate, and provides a subjective feeling with supportive objective evidence. It is not only the patient's brain wave pattern, induced by the healer, which can be assessed, but also his electrical skin resistance (a measure of arousal) and the electrical impulses associated with muscle tension.

After a successful healing session, the machines showed the patient to be more relaxed and at the same time more wide awake and better able to respond to emergencies. In other words, he or she achieves a state where the body can most effectively heal itself. The so-called deep psycho-physical relaxation response, (the very opposite of the flight-or-fight response to stress), has been shown to have extremely beneficial effects on health.[3] First described by Walter Hess in 1957, the physiological correlates include:

—decrease in oxygen consumption;

—reduction in carbon dioxide elimination;

—reduction in: heart rate, respiratory rate, blood pressure, blood lactate, muscle tone and blood cortisone levels.

The unusual brain wave pattern (labelled by Cade as 'State Five) is associated not only with deep relaxation but with bilateral symmetry of brain function, which he claims seems to be central to health control in general.

In conclusion, I think we can now say that the reaction between healer and patient does seem to impose certain beneficial and physiologically measurable patterns. The conclusions so far attained through biofeedback research have recently gained some unexpected support from another research group. Dr Joe Navach, M.D. who has been studying the Auricular Cardiac Reflex (an autonomic or supposedly involuntary function), made some startling discoveries with a new machine designed to record the reflex. Made by NASA and acquired at enormous expense, it is a masterpiece of sensitive technology. It was a shock to find that, as Dr Navach claims, the person working the machine can affect the reading and can 'think' a positive Auricular Cardiac Reflex onto the patient being tested.[4] In other words, if the machine operator is a healer (a fact of which he may be totally unconscious) the results will quickly show up on sensitive instruments; this can lead to horrible complications for those who want to make purely objective measurements!

Bibliography

1. Fulder, Stephen and Monro, Robin. *The Status of Complementary Medicine in the United Kingdom.* Threshold Foundation, 1981
2. Cade, C. Maxwell and Coxhead, Nona. *The Awakened Mind.*

Wildwood House, London, 1980.

Note: Biofeedback is a relatively new and very complex field and it is necessary to point out that there is some disagreement amongst the researchers. I have not, unfortunately, been able to trace published material, but Lee Sannella and Jean Millay are amongst those doing valuable research in the United States.

3. Benson, Herbert. *The Relaxation Response.* Fount Paperbacks, 1977.
4. Novach, J. H. 1980. 'Infra-red photo pulse sensor and doppler investigation of the autonomic vascular system.' Seventh German-Latin Congress of Acupuncture and Auricular Therapy, Palma de Mallorca, Spain.

3. Healing and Wholeness

I would like to explore more fully the idea of 'tuning in' to 'vibrations', good or bad—but in so doing I shall have to enlarge the concept of healing. The physicists now tell us that we are part of a universe that is not nearly as clearly defined as we perceive it. Fritjof Capra[1] states:

> In classical physics, the mass of an object has always been associated with an indestructible material substance, with some 'stuff' of which all things were thought to be made. Relativity theory showed that mass has nothing to do with any stuff, but is a form of energy. Energy, however, is a dynamic quantity associated with activity, or with processes. The fact that the mass of a particle is equivalent to a certain amount of energy means that the particle can no longer be seen as a static object, but has to be conceived as a dynamic pattern, a process involving the energy which manifests itself as the particle's mass . . . In modern physics, the universe is thus experienced as a dynamic, inseparable whole which always includes the observer in an essential way.

This gives some weight to the very simple view that I hold that everything we can see, touch or feel is energy vibrating at some rate and that, theoretically, it should be possible to pick up the vibrations of not only obviously living matter, but of everything on the planet, from apparently inert matter upwards. This would include not only humans and animals, but plant life and even the mineral elements of the earth itself.

Obviously, all is not well with our planet and the life on it. Look not only at the numbers crowding our hospitals; look at the erosion of the earth itself. About 30 per cent of all global land is now reckoned to be desert, and this includes more than nine million square miles which were once productive land and are now man-made deserts. These are still growing at the alarming rate of 60,000 square kilometres per year. To put it into perspective, the remaining food-producing land in the world today is about thirteen million square kilometres[2] The wonderful corn growing areas of North America are apparently being reduced to desert at the rate of an area greater than the county of Yorkshire every single year.

This regrettable prodigality is emulated in this country which can ill afford to lose a square inch of its valuable agricultural land. Lincolnshire top soil can be seen on a windy day simply blowing into the sea, and certain areas have already been reduced to such an infertile state that they will not be of use for many generations. If we define healing not merely as curing symptoms but as making and becoming more whole, of bringing out the full potential, then we can include all life forms, and even the earth itself in the category of things worthy of our attention.

This is not as strange as it may sound. We all know of those who have a way with animals. We talk of someone having green fingers, and many craftsmen would appear to have a feel for the medium in which they work, be it wood or stone. They are, if you like, peculiarly in tune with the particular forms of life or the materials with which they work.

While working with stone is not my *métier* and animals may not be yours, we nonetheless all have this capacity to tune in to some extent in some field. More importantly, we are not using anything supernatural or odd. We are merely using our own senses, but at a level which we are not fully aware of and do not properly recognize. Many of the bushmen or tribal peoples who can 'know' in advance when strangers are approaching explain their knowledge in terms of smell or sight. Patently they are not using their senses in a way that fits into our conceptual framework, but they are equally obviously using their senses in some way that we do not understand. We dimly recognize these possibilities in the symbols we use in speech. We say, 'I see' when someone has explained something to us; we talk of 'smelling a rat'. In neither of these cases do we see or smell in the normal way but I maintain that we are nonetheless using our basic senses at a different level.

So we can use our physical senses in some way to perceive the non-physical. We can use them to tune in with or become more aware of the world and life around us. But what happens next?

The Healing Energy

To return to humans, it would seem that tuning in can enable a person to become more open to help in any form. But the full picture is more complex. If the expression 'in tune' has some reality, how about 'good vibrations'? If we can tune in, then it should be possible to set up responsive vibrations which resonate beneficially. This is a hypothesis, but resonance is a simple concept in physics, which at its simplest means that by transmitting on the same frequency we can reinforce and increase the strength of the original wave.

To put it a different way, when a healer 'tunes in' to a patient, some form of energy seems to be transmitted for the patient's benefit. Two more problems promptly arise: What sort of energy is this?; and what is meant by the statement 'for the patient's benefit'? There are plenty of people who will give you an opinion on the first question. There are those who will refer to Odic force or cosmic energy or 'chi' or electro-magnetism. There are those who say it comes from God. (But then, arguably, all energy comes from God.)

The energy involved in healing is not fully understood, but then neither are numerous other forms of energy. Electricity is perhaps one of the best known forms and we have observed it and learnt to generate, transform and harness it. We still do not know exactly what it is, however, and events in 1979 in Fishpond, a village in Dorset, showed that it may not be as closely under our control as we thought. Residents of the village became extremely perturbed when after the erection of power cables over the village there was an upsurge of various forms of malaise. The electricity board concerned hotly denied the possibility of a 'leak' being responsible, but the fact remains that there is a television film showing a procession of villagers carrying strip lighting bulbs in their hands which lit up as the procession moved through the area, despite the fact that these strips were not connected to any cables.

We may not understand the healing energy, but it appears to be available for human use. As a non-scientist, I am not clear about a number of things. The term 'healing energy', denoting a special quality of energy may well be misleading. The ability to tune in and resonate suggests that we can operate on a myriad of frequencies, working through existing forms. I suggest that individuals and groups of people can transform and employ energy of various frequencies to bring about physical change in their fellow humans, animals and plant life. Analogies are necessarily inadequate, but it is obvious that the very high voltage available in the national grid system must be modified to suit household equipment, and I maintain that some human beings, so-called healers, bring about some similar result for their patients. It would probably therefore be more appropriate to say 'the many energy frequencies which healers can transform for their patients' or some such long-winded phrase; however, as this is cumbersome I shall stick to the shorter if slightly inaccurate label 'healing energy'.

It would appear that the healer's state of mind is probably important in enabling him to act as a transformer, but that the energy does have a reality apart from the 'mental' link or 'tuning in' measured by multi-channel encephalographs. Professor Justa Smith, an enzymologist at Buffalo University, studied the effect of healing upon enzymes by exposing solutions of trypsin to the hands of the Hungarian healer, Oscar Estavani. He found that the solutions' level of activity could be increased by 100 per cent when held by Estavani for an hour. Even more remarkably, a jar of enzyme solution which had been damaged by previous exposure to ultra-violet light and had lost 30 per cent activity in consequence had its level restored to normal by being held for 20 minutes by the healer.[3] It should be added that these experiments were carried out during the vacation. When repeated in the bustle of term-time when Estavani was also under emotional stress, nothing happened. This failure does not invalidate the original experiments, but it does show that the healer's state of mind probably affects his ability to act as a transformer.

It would be a help if this healing energy could be satisfactorily measured. Solutions of trypsin could also have their level of activity increased by 100 per cent by exposing them to a strong magnetic field. However, when a magnetometer was used to determine whether Estavani naturally produced a magnetic field between his hands, a nil reading was obtained. This suggests that there must be something more than a magnetic field involved, although this may be part of the mechanism involved.

Great excitement was generated by the discovery of Kirlian photography, which very convincingly claims to 'photograph' energy fields around any living matter. These 'photographs' are taken without any light source and result from electric discharges between an object and an electrode. The Kirlian process was used to test healers and patients before and after treatment. The patient's 'energy field' was found to be considerably strengthened and photographs of healers' hands while they were working supposedly showed streams of energy emanating from the finger-tips or palms.[4] This research started in the USSR,[5] but it is now being actively pursued both here and in the United States. The process indicates that our energy pattern can be profoundly affected by fatigue, exertion, state of mind and, of course, illness. Most important of all, perhaps, is the contention that imminent disease shows up in the photographed energy pattern before any physical symptoms appear. If this can be confirmed, then Kirlian photography will be an inestimably useful 'early warning' system, allowing us to take preventive measures in good time.

Kirlian photography is unfortunately far from being established as yet, however, because the processes involved have given cause for doubts to arise as to whether the Kirlian process is merely an artefact.[6] The validity of the colours supposedly recorded may be in doubt as they could be merely the result of the Kirlian processes on colour film. It seems, however, that the evidence for the process' capacity to record some energy field is overwhelming. The scientist's contention that this energy cannot be 'psychic' energy worries me not a whit as I have always been sure that healing energy can manifest physically, even if it is not yet measurable.

Leaving aside the problem of defining and measuring the energies involved, what do we mean by saying they are available for the patient's benefit? When someone comes to me for help, it may be perfectly obvious that his hands are stiff and swollen with arthritis; or he may tell me that his doctor has diagnosed such and such a complaint. As a healer, to whom most patients only come as a result of failure to respond to orthodox treatment, I assume that some unknown factor is inhibiting the patient's response. If I can tune in to the patient (as demonstrated by the encephalograph experiments), I can respond to the areas, both physical and non-physical, which are not working in harmony. I may not consciously recognize what I am doing, but energy will be transformed for the patient. The patient in his turn may have no conscious knowledge of what is wrong with him. The pain in his back may be due to an undiagnosed kidney complaint or he may not recognize the psychological factors that contribute to his all-too-real ulcer. Some aspects of the subconscious mind which is responsible for the involuntary organization of the body will be aware of what is going on, however, and will be able to use the healing energy constructively.

We Are More Than Just Our Bodies
The introduction of the conscious and the unconscious and of the inter-play between physiological and psychological factors may still cause some people, who believe in the purely mechanistic theory of disease, to shift uneasily in their chairs. But we are undoubtedly extremely complex beings. We have a body and brain, a mind and emotions. Thanks to the work of Freud and Jung, it is now recognized that we have a subconscious as well. We possess other non-physical features, but it is difficult to map these out, not least because those who have tried to do so in the past have used different terminology and held to different emotive beliefs. 'Higher', 'lower' and 'inner' selves mean different things to different people, as do the words 'soul' and 'spirit'. I shall avoid these arguments for the moment, and merely state that we are all obviously very much more than just our bodies.

All these aspects of ourselves—our mind, our emotions and subconscious, let alone the rest—exist and express themselves through our bodies. Disturbance to any one level of our being can easily upset the delicate balance and result in bodily malfunction. Doctors are becoming increasingly aware of this and the term 'wholistic (or holistic) medicine' is no mere *cliché*.

The Psychosomatic Factor
The word psychosomatic admits the link between psyche and body and this link is already recognized as a contributor to a number of ailments. Ulcers are perhaps the best known examples of this, but one can reel off many others from asthma to cancer. What seems to happen is that emotional 'dis-ease' (stress or anxiety) results in a mal-

functioning in some way of the body's normal repairing and immunity system, making it prone to illness or break-down. The Simontons, who run a highly successful cancer clinic in the U.S.A. are some of the many both in and out of the medical world who are convinced that emotional and mental states play a significant role both in susceptibility to disease, including cancer, and in recovery from the disease.[7] If the integrated system of mind, body and emotions which constitutes the whole person is not working together towards healthiness, then purely physical interventions may not succeed. Ideally, two things seem to be required. The patient should try to identify and understand the cause of stress. Secondly, the supposedly involuntary processes should somehow or other be encouraged to do their job properly.

Biofeedback research has already shown us that a number of supposedly involuntary processes can be brought under our conscious control. Max Cade's work has clearly indicated that if people can learn to control and counteract the physiological manifestations of stress, numerous other complaints and illnesses can be alleviated. Sometimes, the reduction of stress is itself enough to remove some physical symptom. In others, it seems to allow the body to respond to treatment which had previously proved inexplicably ineffective.

Cade is not only concerned with teaching control of the physical correlates of stress. He is especially interested in states of awareness. The two go hand in hand as those who have learnt to relax properly whenever necessary also report that they can now cope much better with the situations which had previously caused stress. The incredibly sensitive and close link between our body, emotions, mind and subconscious is central to healing which aims not just at alleviating a physical symptom but at restoring wholeness. The physical symptom which has driven the patient to seek help will of course receive attention, but the healing energy can reach out to any other cause, be it another unknown physiological imbalance or some psychological disturbance which may, unrecognized, be the reason for the persistent resistance of the physical symptom.

Bibliography

1. Capra, Fritjof. *The Tao of Physics*. Fontana, 1976.
2. Precise figures vary, but for current assessments of the destruction of productive land, see the following:
   Eckholm, Eric. *Down to Earth*. Pluto Press, 1982.
   Tolba, Mostafa K. *Development Without Destruction*. Tycooly, Dublin, 1982.
   United Nations Environment Programme's Report: *The Earth Environment*, 1972-82.
3. A number of people are studying healers' effects on enzymes. I

have discussed their work with some of them but I do not know of any published material. Professor Justa Smith's experiment is quoted by Dr Ian Pearce in his article 'The Healer Priest in Modern Times' in *New Humanity* December-January 1981-82 No. 42.

4. Moss, Thelma. *Galaxies of Life.* Gordon and Breach, 1973.

5. Ostrander, Sheila and Schroeder, Lynn. *Psychic Discoveries Behind the Iron Curtain.* Sphere Books, 1976.
   see also:
   Gris, Henry and Dick, William. *New Soviet Psychic Discoveries.* Sphere Books, 1980.

6. Tiller, William A. *New Scientists,* 25 April 1979.
   Boyers, D. G. and Tiller, William A. *Journal of Applied Physics,* Vol. 44 No. 7, July 1973.

7. Simonton, O. Carl, Matthews-Simonton, Stephanie and Creighton, James L. *Getting Well Again.* Bantam Books, 1980.

4. First Experience of 'Laying on Hands'

My own experience with healing began as a spontaneous activity during the French campaign of May 1940 and was entirely brought about by the lack of medical facilities in my unit. Horrified that men were being wounded and were without the comfort of anaesthetics or trained medical personnel, I felt impelled to put my hands on them. I did not have a great deal of time to think about what I was doing as the pressure forcing us back to the coast demanded all our concentration. It was only later, therefore, that I could feel real surprise at the results: haemorrhaging had been arrested; we had no morphine, but when I had put a hand (or two if I could spare them) on a wounded man, pain had started to ebb immediately; the effects of shock and exhaustion seemed to have been minimized.

The results were remarkable and persistent and to me both fascinating and extraordinary. It was not something which I could ignore. In the heat of war, I felt a duty to pursue the matter and used my hands whenever necessary. This happened in various circumstances, including the bombing of Britain, accidents during training during the years 1940-42 and thereafter in an infantry division in North Africa and in Italy.

Reactions in My Hands and From the Patient
I discovered that both I and the person I was treating could feel a variety of reactions. Most people reported a marked change of temperature. Normally they felt heat greater than one would expect from the mere touch of a human hand, but sometimes they would tell me they had experienced intense cold, almost as if a cold wind was blowing on the area I was touching. Sometimes the pain was so great that the patients could not bear being touched and I would have to hold my hand a little away from the wound, but the temperature change could still be felt. Occasionally, they would report a tingling feeling like pins and needles, or throbbing. Others felt that the pain intensified initially and then diffused and seemed to drain away. Sensations

recorded less frequently have included a feeling of pressure as though the healer were leaning on the patient when, in fact, there may not have been any physical contact, and indeed very recently one patient exclaimed about the pressure on her chest when my hands were lightly touching her back. Since the war years, I have compared notes with thousands of people and these various reactions seem to be widely shared. Some healers can feel in their hands what is going on. Others feel nothing with their hands but can sense what is happening, sometimes by feeling the pain or illness in their own bodies. This happens to me on occasions. It can be extremely awkward if you are sitting at a dinner party and you develop a very painful knee or an appalling headache which you may be picking up from your neighbour.

Locating by Following a Line of Reaction on the Body

During the war, my healing activities, which of necessity were carried out in my spare time, were mostly concerned with helping the wounded, so that it was usually obvious where I should put my hands. Sometimes I would find that reaction to my hands was not limited to the wounded area and by moving my hands slowly and gently around, I could find a line of reaction away from the wound. This could be helpful in the case of shrapnel wounds as I could trace the damaged tissue when the offending bits of shell had lodged themelves in the body some inches from the point of entry. Using my hands as detectors, I found that I could scan the body and could find other areas of pain or damage—pulled or torn muscles, strained backs, fractured bones and the like. Increasingly, I found that the back seemed to be particularly sensitive even when there was no obvious damage to that area. I would find that I would have to keep my hands for a long time on some point on a patient's back before the reaction faded and frequently the patient would report that a symptom elsewhere, such as a headache, pain in the knee, a numb finger, would disappear. I began to wonder if there was a relationship.

Response of Supposedly Nervous Disorders

On occasion, I tried to help men who had not been physically wounded but were suffering from nervous exhaustion and various forms of tension which were generally summed up as battle fatigue. Very frequently I seemed to be able to help them so that they could go back into action very quickly without recourse to prolonged psychiatric treatment. As I did not know what to do when confronted with someone who had no overt injury, I would merely scan with my hands until I found a spot where the patient or I or both found a reaction. In every case, I found, amongst other reactions, a precise point in the spine at the level of the fourth and fifth thoracic vertebrae. This happened so consistently that I could not accept it as coincidence. Could there be specific physical areas related to nervous disorders? This seemingly extraordinary hypotheses became for me inescapable fact when, over the years, I found that the majority of patients suffering from nervous disorders, including major psychoses such as schizophrenia and obsession, have a lesion, whether painful or not, at the same point.

Central Nervous System as the Bridge

The word 'psychosomatic', recognizing the interaction between the 'psyche' and the 'soma' (body) gave me an inkling in those early days. If we are not just our physical bodies but a multitude of non-physical characteristics which have to express themselves through the body, there must be some point of interaction. The main conductor of energy up and down the body is the central nervous system, which is housed in the skull and the spine *en route* to the consumer unit, which might be a muscle, organ, gland or any other part of the body. It is my belief that it is this central nervous system, housed in the spine, which is the main area of interaction between our physical and non-physical attributes.

In emphasizing the significance for me personally of the spinal cord and its associated neural network, I am in no way turning a blind eye to that important part of the central nervous system which is supraterritorial—the brain. This is the happy hunting ground of psychologists and hypnotherapists who, in their turn, give only indirect attention to the rest of the nervous system. Each to his own natural bent! My main purpose is to stress the importance of the central nervous system and hence the spine to both our physical *and non-physical* health.

5. The Physical Importance of the Spine

Once the war was over, I found that the feeling in my hands and the response they could call forth did not go away. I remained in the army until 1959 and, increasingly, my spare time was taken up with trying to help people with their various illnesses and complaints which were of course no longer restricted to war damage. Time and time again, when scanning the body with my hands, I would find a point of reaction in the back.

Osteopaths, chiropractors and those concerned with orthopaedics are already familiar with the importance of the spine in relation to a multitude of physical complaints not obviously connected with the back. I had certainly not discovered anything new. Hippocrates who lived from 460 to 377 B.C. and wrote over 70 books, including one entitled *Manipulation and Importance to Good Health* urged his followers to 'get knowledge of the spine, for this is the requisite for many diseases.' A little later, Galen (130-200 A.D.) was given the title 'Prince of Physicians' after he cured the paralysed right arm of the Roman, Eudemus, by treating his neck. He also told his students to look to the nervous system as the key to maximum health. Despite its long history, this knowledge has not always found favour and I still have to stress the importance of the spine, even at the purely physical level, as many people overlook it completely and may indeed hotly deny its importance.

Neurological Effect on Pathology

Before going on to talk about the spine, I must say a little about the nervous system which serves every organ and every limb and is vital to the proper funcitioning of virtually every single aspect of our bodies. While many factors can impair health, disturbances of any kind which produce abnormal fluctuations in the pattern of nerve impulses can lead to or aggravate disease. Disturbance of nerve impulses can have a number of causes, ranging from degenerative conditions to compression (or what in lay language I call 'trapping') of nerves.

Pressure on the nervous system at any point, be it the spine , in a joint or in congested muscle tissue, will have a detrimental effect on the consumer unit served by the nerves in question. What is more, in certain circumstances, almost any component of the nervous system may directly or indirectly cause reactions within any other component by means of reflex mediation, so that it is not only the unit directly served by a 'trapped' nerve that is affected.

As everyone knows, the spinal column is the great central pipeline for the nervous system. Because of the way we are made and our insistence on standing upright, the back is subject to a great deal of strain and stress and the opportunities for pressure on nerves at the points where they leave the spine between the vertebrae is unfortunately enormous. I am not by any means claiming that every single illness or discomfort has a direct connection with the spine, but I do find that it is an area which is worth very careful attention.

X-rays and Electro-myelograms

On many occasions, I have been assured by patients that X-rays disclose no faults in the spine and yet the symptoms persist. The trouble is that X-ray cannot show nerves. Healing techniques have shown time and time again that what appears perfect, either on X-ray or other systems of medical examination, can in fact still be producing pressure on the nervous system, leading to symptoms elsewhere in the body. (Conversely, structural faults in the spine do not necessarily produce a symptom through the related part of the nervous system. It is possible for someone to live painlessly and problem-free for years with a malformed or structurally damaged spine, provided the nerve pathways operate freely. I well remember an old man in our village who was badly distorted. Even his head was malformed. Yet he lived into his eighties and remained amazingly fit and pain-free all his days.)

As nerves do not show up on X-ray it is very difficult to corroborate my analyses except circumstantially. True, nerve compression can be measured by electro-myelograms which show that nerve conduction is altered when reflex, power or sensation (or all three) are affected, but this only goes part of the way and, in any case, is only available at specialist level. A healer with diagnostic ability can trace the trouble very much more quickly and completely without any danger of side effects. I will go into more detail about this in Chapter 7.

Relationships Between Areas in the Spine and Symptoms Elsewhere

Consistent experience through the years has led me to associate a variety of symptoms with areas in the spine. I must stress again that to claim that the spine is important is not to claim that it is the only factor in disease; far from it. I am only too conscious of bacteriological illness, viruses and organic and cellular malfunction, and I have already emphasized the part which minds and emotions can play. We all know, however, that while there may be a virulent brand of 'flu around, not everyone succumbs. It would appear that if the body's natural immunizing and repairing functions fail, there must be additional underlying reasons for them to do so. In many cases, it would seem that one such reason is provided by impediments to the nerves controlling the appropriate part of the body.

I would maintain that certain symptoms are nearly always related to the spine. In others, nerves in the spinal area indicated can be a strong contributory factor, but are not inevitably involved. Unfortunately for those of us who like life to be simple, there is very seldom one cause and one symptom, and in any diagnosis vast permutations are possible! It is always worth looking to the nervous system, however, if a given symptom is refusing to respond to normal medical treatment.

In general terms, varicose veins, troublesome feet, sciatica, prostate trouble in men, period pains in women and even, on occasion, failure to conceive, can all be said to have a close relationship with the lumbar region. This area can also have an effect on the kidneys and, in some cases, migraine. I have found the area at the base of the neck (from the seventh cervical vertebra to the second and third thoracic vertebrae) seems to be indicated in many headache cases and also with loss of movement or discomfort in the shoulders, arms and hands. A few cases of *angina pectoris* proved to be partially related to the first and second thoracic vertebrae. I have known a number of exciting instances where the release of nerves in this area has removed indefinitely the symptoms of angina and enabled the sufferer to go back to his normal way of life without drugs. The cervical and high thoracic areas in fact seem to be to the nervous system what Crewe Junction was to the old railway system of Britain. This area seems to have a positive connection with vision as well as hearing, sinuses, catarrh and tinnitus (noises in the ears), amongst other things.

Osteopathy and Chiropractic Neuro-spinology
Many a patient who has appeared with stomach trouble or a pain in the knee has looked at me incredulously when I have turned my attention to the spine. My approach has always been empirical, and I soon found that even if I was deluded, I was not on my own! Many other individuals and groups have become convinced of the relevance of the spine to symptoms elsewhere. Both osteopaths and chiropractors recognize its importance, though they vary in the emphasis they place on it. Their published findings, as far as I have access to them, tally with my discoveries on many points, though not on all of them. (The areas of disagreement are proof to me that more research needs to be done on this subject.)

Therapies

Osteopaths and chiropractors amongst others realize the importance of impeded nerve pathways or, as I put it, trapped nerves, and they do something about it. The healer who comes across the same problem then has to decide what to do. For many years. I merely laid my hands on the appropriate point. This seemed to do the trick on many occasions which indicates that physiological changes can be brought about merely by the healing energy, but at least for me it was a slow process. Therapies of various sorts can speed up the treatment. It is sensible, therefore, to pass the patient on to someone who can untrap the nerves. This is what I did for a long time if the effect of the laying on of hands proved incomplete. Over the years, however, I have evolved very gentle techniques myself. Without doing anything violent and using mainly the patient's own weight and breathing, I can help them to correct the problem. I spend a great deal of my time lecturing and teaching on this subject and I would like to sound a very strong warning note that manipulation of any sort must be treated with great care and circumspection and remains the field of the specialist.

6. Bridges Between the Physical and the Non-physical

If we really are more than just our physical bodies and have various psychological, emotional and spiritual factors in our make-up which have to manifest through the body and can affect our bodily health, there must be a physical cross-over point. The reactions I found in soldiers suffering from battle fatigue first gave me a hint. Forty years later, sheer empiricism has convinced me that the most important physical bridge is the central nervous system housed in the spine.

Perhaps at this point I should say a little more about the complexities of the nervous system which may help in making sense of the interplay between physical and non-physical functions. I do not know the precise mechanism by which healing is transmitted either to physical or non-physical problems, but the autonomic nerves as well as the spinal nerves themselves probably play a part! The autonomic nerves control the activities of the blood vessels, secretory glands (including the hormonal or endocrine glands) and the viscera. This autonomic system is constantly at work and may be likened to the administrative branches of an army. Its activities do not normally obtrude into consciousness. The autonomic nerves are arranged in networks and ganglia strung up and down each side of the vertebral column along its entire length. Autonomic ganglia have also been located in many parts of the brain itself. As these autonomic nerves are interconnected into a 'system of administration', at the same time connecting with the spinal cord and brain centres, it is not difficult to see how it is that healing techniques applied along the sides of the spine could have remote effects on cerebral activities controlled by brain centres within the skull itself. Such functions and activities include not only such things as sight, hearing, sense of balance and speech but also emotional feelings and creative thought.

The Spine and Non-Physical Problems

To insist upon the importance of the central nervous system in the spine as the link between the physical and the non-physical is not to say that everyone with a sore back is in fact really suffering from some deep-seated psychological emotional or spiritual problem, but it does mean that almost everyone with a deep-seated problem of this nature will have an area in the spine that is a potential trouble-maker. Even if there is no pain in the back, there will nearly always be some reaction from the healer's hands at certain points in the spine. If the physical manifestations can be alleviated, the patient has a much better chance of coping with the non-physical problem and of responding thereafter to more orthodox forms of treatment.

The Spine and Nervous Disorders

The interval between the fourth and fifth thoracic vetebrae seems to me to be vitally connected with all nervous disorders, from battle fatigue (as I then knew it) to schizophrenia and obsession. I have found many other specific areas related to non-physical problems. Those suffering from insomnia or from lethargy, for example, usually seem to have a lesion between the second and third thoracic vertebrae, and I have found that the area around the sixth and seventh vertebrae is similarly related to allergies, many of which are suspected of having a psychological basis. Treatment at this point frequently alleviates asthma, hay fever, nervous eczema, skin trouble and even occasionally stammering as well as easily upset stomachs, including cases where the patient displays every symptom of an ulcerated stomach except the ulcer. In addition, the patient seems to receive help to live with the probably unrecognized psychological problems. In many cases, however, care has to be taken, as the physical symptoms may well be a valuable warning of a more serious malaise requiring treatment.

In some cases, healing can relieve physical symptoms on all occasions except when psychological needs demand their return as a shield. One girl with asthma, for example, found that her symptoms had completely disappeared—except when she was at her parents' home! It seemed that some psychological stress in the home environment demanded the protection of her asthma. I subsequently discovered that though she hated riding, she was expected to go out hunting with her father and this caused her considerable distress.

Having said all this, I must add that it is too simple to say that by treating the back one is eradicating some non-physical problem. But the appropriate point in the spine is the gateway, if you like, for energy to flow into the body for use either at the physical or the non-physical level. Better still, the energy can go both ways.

The Eastern Approach and the Chakras

The idea of 'gateways' was and is well known to many of the oriental disciplines. In India, they are called 'chakras'. Their concept is perhaps nearer to what I am trying to express, since they do not distinguish as we do between 'medicine' and philosophy or spirituality. These chakras could be considered as the gateways into and between different parts of the physical body and between levels of consciousness. In our terms, this would include the concept that at certain points in the body a physical defect could lead to psychological stress and vice versa. There are many beautiful representations of the chakras which are shown as symbols on the body. Usually they are shown on the front of the body but sometimes a line is shown connecting each chakra to a point in the spine. The spine is very important to oriental thought but the lack of distinction between the physical and non-physical features makes it easy for them to see the whole body as playing a part in all the aspects of man, including his spirituality.

I find this a helpful concept with healing. The spine is of vital importance, but it is not the only bridge since the rest of the body can also be seen as functioning at different levels simultaneously. There are many chakras, but most disciplines select about seven particularly important ones, though opinion varies on which are the most significant. I find nine which seem to be crucial to well-being. The first two are shown on the cranium and seem to be concerned with aspiration, perception, interpretation and understanding. The third is on the throat, the centre for communication. If you consider that not only the vocal cords, but the nerves serving the arms and hands with which we also communicate are situated in this area, the concept ties in quite neatly. Traditional laying on of hands within the Christian church concentrates on these areas and I would suspect that this implies an instinctive awareness, or indeed the ancient if forgotten knowledge of these important gateways. The fourth is placed over the heart, the centre of emotions, of love and of hate. Language points to our awareness of emotional well-being as vital to physical health and we talk of heartache or a shaft to the heart. The fifth lies on the solar plexus, the centre of energy. Again, we talk of a blow to the solar plexus when a shock drains our energy.

The sixth chakra is what I would call the 'city cleansing centre', situated at the level of navel, kidney, liver and spleen—the organs of filtration, detoxification, recirculation, elimination and insulation. I find the latter very important. In the same way that mankind has a problem with nuclear waste which can be dealt with only by effective insulation because currently it cannot be transformed or eliminated, individuals have to cope with damaging materials of both physical and non-physical types. If I find a reaction over the spleen, this may mean that energy is needed at a purely physical level. But energy may also be valuable at a psychological level of understanding of the spleen as the 'insulator' of any problem which cannot currently be resolved or eliminated.

The next chakra is below the navel and I find it to be associated with courage and determination and what you might call 'fire'. We refer to a 'lack of guts' when someone's courage has evaporated. The sacral or sexual centre is of enormous importance, not only at the obvious level of reproduction, but also as the home of a driving force which can be available at other creative levels, if successfully transformed or sublimated. The ninth chakra at the base of the spine is much more mysterious but appears to be a basic element of the life force, known in the East as the home of the Kundalini serpent. The complexities of the chakras are unfortunately outside the scope of this book, but it is the failure to handle any or all these energies successfully and use them in some other creative endeavour that can lead to the problems of repression and consequent cries for help. Almost invariably, I find in such people spinal lesions influencing the effective interplay of energy between the appropriate centres.

Interplay and Transformation of Energy

The idea of sublimating or transforming energy is not unfamiliar. Recognizing but wishing to discourage the direct expression of the very powerful adolescent sex drive, public schools advocated cold baths (a sort of fire extinguisher) and long runs, thereby converting the sexual energy into strenuous athletic activity. This is a very basic example of sublimation, but we are familiar, too, with the idea of emotional energy being transformed into creative expression. Some superb music and literature has been written as a direct result of the agony or ecstasy of a love-affair. We seem to be made up of many energies which permeate the body through many specific 'gateways'; each of the energies being capable of actually flowing up, down and around the body. If there is a 'block' at some level, the energy can bypass it and find expression at another level. Alternatively, if the gateway is not working properly, the energy may drain away.

The blocks and problems that occur can be likened to the plumbing system of a bath. If you turn on the tap and no water comes out, either the tap is blocked or there is something wrong futher back up the system. Equally troublesome is a tap that will not turn off and wastes all your hot water. If you lose the bath plug, the bath will not fill up at all as the water drains away immediately, and a blocked wastepipe will cause the bath to overflow and flood the bathroom. In the same way the faults or blocks in the 'gateways', be it in the input system or output system of the energy flow, can cause trouble. Our language expresses some idea of this as we use expressions such as 'I feel drained' when energy is lacking or, 'she was bubbling over' of someone in good spirits and full of vitality. I am convinced that a free but controllable flow of energy, whether this means removing a block, adjusting a gateway or ensuring that the bypass system works properly, is vital to good health

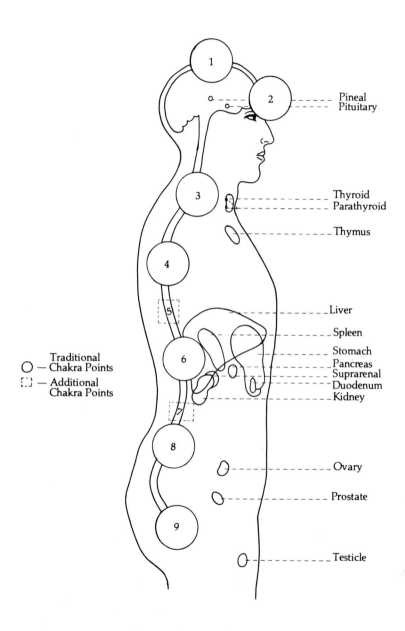

Figure 3. Suggested chakra system.

and the full enjoyment of life. My own suggestions of the principal functional levels and gateways are shown in the chart opposite.

These flows of energy are very real to me. I can feel them and on occasion see them. They have been known for thousands of years in the East and indeed some of the religious training concentrates on this flow and transformation of energy for use at different levels. They are and have been reported consistently and persistently by multitides of people throughout the millenia and in all parts of the world. Such corroboration makes it necessary to entertain at least a hypothesis that such things may in fact exist, though they have not yet been verified by instrumentation. As we have now developed instuments that can pick up radio waves, cosmic rays and hundreds of other energy frequencies unknown only a few decades ago, I have great hopes that appropriate instrumentation will soon be found.

If and when devices for recording these energies are found, it may be possible to ascertain whether my theory that the chakras tie in with the endocrine system has any validity. I have long suspected that the mysterious and complicated ductless glands play a vital role in the transformation of energy and I now find that others have come to a similar conclusion. Dr Shafica Karagulla, a neuro-psychiatrist with an outstanding medical and psychiatric background of research and practice in four countries including Britain and the United States, set herself the task of researching the creative frontiers of the mind and what she calls 'Higher Sense Perception.'[2] Amongst the multitude of people she studied, she mentions 'Diane' who could see energy patterns from which she could diagnose the condition of a patient. In every case her findings were confirmed by medical diagnosis. Diane sees the energy as vortices, and is particularly interested in seven of the major ones which she claims are directly related to the ductless glands. As the studies of her work in the endocrine clinic of a large New York hospital showed, what she saw in these major vortices certainly described exactly the condition of the appropriate gland. The chiropractor and fomer President of the Radionics Association, David Tansley, also suggests a connection between the chakras and the endocrine system.[3]

Auras and Higher Energy Bodies

The interplay of energies permeating the body can also be seen, felt and described (though once again not yet adequately measured by instrumentation) in a further form. Many people see or feel the so-called aura, a force field often seen as a colour or colours permeating and surrounding the physical body. The halo in old religious paintings is thought to be representative of this aura and indeed many Byzantine paintings show the 'halo' extending not just round the head but, round the whole body. According to which colours they see and the quality of the colour (bright, dull or opaque) many people with this gift can give a very accurate analysis of the physical and often the mental and emotional states of the person concerned.

Although science cannot yet measure this field or fields of energy, W. J. Kilner, a physician and X-ray specialist at St Thomas' hospital at the beginning of this century, was certain that they exist, and developed a screen through which these fields could be made visible to the eye. Many people found that by using the screen initially their vision developed and they could then see auras without its help.

I say that science cannot yet measure these fields, but some startling discoveries have been made recently by a Rumanian called Dumitrescu[4]. His work clearly demonstrates that around the body, extending to about two or three inches, is a highly important electrically cognisant layer which he terms 'the proximal electric medium'. It is mostly ionic mixed with water vapour and it is very adherent to the skin surface. Very important electrical exchanges take place in this zone between the body and the zone itself, and presumably further electrical exchanges take place between the zone and the so-called outer electrical medium within which we all move. This may well be a breakthrough to a scientific understanding of the aura, at least in its relevance to physical well-being.

Shafica Karagulla, amongst many others, claims that there are three distinct interpenetrating fields of energy within the total aura. One of these which may share properties with the proximal electric medium is closely related to the physical. Any disease or malfunction in the physical body can be seen in its energy field and indeed changes in the energy field seem to precede reactions in the physical body as it can be seen to be depleted or affected in some way *before* physical symptoms appear. I and many others would claim not only that it is possible to perceive this field and to read information from it, but that by applying healing to it, the physical body can then be affected. The same goes for the other two fields, the emotional and mental.

There are in fact more than three fields, but some people 'see' more than others and give them different names. While some say that we have a 'soul' body, others claim that we have a spiritual *and* a soul body. This is not the place to argue over details, and I would merely suggest that, as complex beings, we have a series of even more refined levels of awareness or frequencies, each of which requires a 'body' or 'field' in which to manifest at the appropriate level.

Conclusion

The unsuspecting healer, when he or she first puts his hands on a patient requesting help, probably does not know what he is in for! I used to put my hands on a patient, endeavouring to help some physical problem. I discovered that I could help psychological problems and that points in the spine were vital in this respect. I then found that I could feel energies leading up and down, as well as places where the flow of energy was blocked or draining away uncontrollably. This would seem to be a very concrete, physical manifestation of a concept known to the orient as the interplay of energy between functional centres. A healer may therefore be restoring the flow or balance of energy, but it is significant that he or she need have no intellectual awareness of exactly what occurs.

The idea of balancing flows of energy is very highly developed in the complex and precise knowledge of acupuncture.[5] Although I have not studied acupuncture in any depth, some of the points which I have found to be useful in restoring energy balance do tie in with acupuncture points, and pressure with the finger-tips (so-called acupressure) can be very helpful. Western medicine is coming to accept not only the empirical evidence for acupuncture but also the reality of the acupuncture points, as treatment through them can be seen to have physiologically measurable consequences. We may be coming closer to an intellectual recognition of the energy flows that I have suggested.

Bibliography

1. *Gray's Anatomy* 35th Edition. Longman 1973.
2. Karagulla, Shafica. *Breakthrough to Creativity.* De Vorss, California, 1967.
3. Tansley, David V. *Subtle Body.* Thames and Hudson, 1977.
4. For this information I am extremely grateful to Dr Julian Kenyon who is currently translating and editing Dumitrescu's work.
5. Lewith, George T. *Acupuncture: Its Place in Western Medical Science*, Thorsons, 1982.

7. Dowsing and Absent Healing

It is all very well to talk about locating problem areas in the spine, or anywhere else for that matter. It can, of course, be done by using the hands to 'scan'; this can be a slow process, however. Both to save time and to obtain more detailed analysis I now use dowsing[1], and find it invaluable.

Tradition of Water Divining
Water divining is probably the best known form of dowsing. It is a capability which has been known of for thousands of years in many parts of the world. Finding water is obviously very useful but a good dowser can do more than that. He should be able to discover the location, depth, direction and rate of flow and mineral content of the water. He should also be able to find out about the geological strata above the water which would enable others to decide on the viability of drilling, and he should know whether the water will then well up of its own accord or whether it will require pumping.

Methods of Dowsing
There are all sorts of methods. Some people use a Y-shaped branch which dips strongly in the diviner's hands when he comes across the object of his search. There is a considerable mystique surrounding dowsing amongst certain groups and you may be told that it is essential to use freshly cut hazel twigs. Personally, I have found that any twig of the right shape or even a bent wire coat-hanger will work equally well. Other people use rods which cross to indicate their message. I normally use a pendulum which, by rotating one way or the other, can indicate positive or negative answers to specific questions.

Application of Dowsing Techniques in Healing
There is relatively little demand for finding water in Britain today but there are many other areas where dowsing techniques can be extremely useful. With the help of the British Society of Dowsers I discovered that

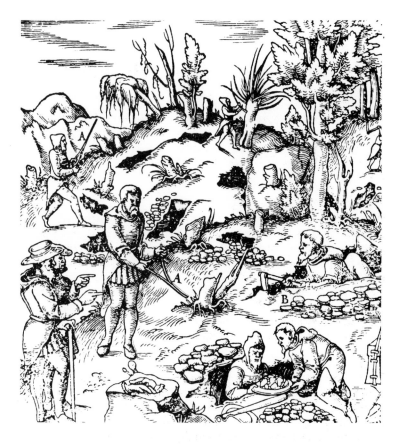

Figure 4. Dowsing for metal — an early German woodcut. From
De Re Metallica by G. Agricola, Basle 1556.

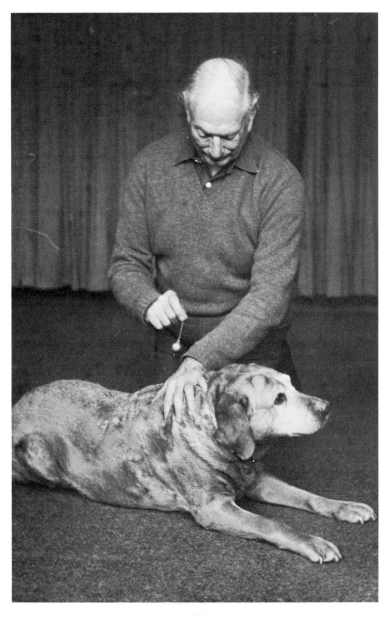

Figure 5. Bruce MacManaway using a pendulum to diagnose illness in a dog.

I could use this faculty and have since applied it to my healing work. For example, I can ask the question 'Is there any pressure on the nervous system of this patient?' If the answer is 'Yes', I can ask a series of detailed questions so that I end up with a comprehensive analysis.

The important thing is to ask *all* the relevant questions. To go back to the water diviner, he would be of little use if he ascertained the position, the depth and the flow but forgot to find out if the water was suitable for human consumption. One of the beautifully simple aids to diagnosis through dowsing is the final question in every instance: should the dowser be asking further questions about this patient? This gives the subconscious the opportunity to draw attention to any relevant material which may not even be consciously known to anyone concerned.

It is up to the intellect to frame the questions. A number of doctors are now finding dowsing a very useful supplement and many of them dowse for themselves. Others, after careful screening, use a lay dowser. It is the doctors, who, with their greater knowledge, frame the necessary questions and the dowser who gives the answers. Over the years, I have built up a system of co-operation with a number of doctors. They test me to begin with, of course. Some doctors in Austria, for example, showed an interest a few years ago and they sent me a series of questions. They knew the answers to some of them but were doubtful about others. I wrote back with my answers and they sent me some more. This little parlour game continued for some time and I wrote endless lists of the only five answers a pendulum can give. (A pendulum can give a straight 'yes', a straight 'no', it can remain neutral or it can give a qualified, half-hearted 'yes' or 'no'. In the last two, I always assume that more questions need to be asked.) Finally, they wrote to me confessing that they had been so surprised by the results that they had had to repeat the experiment a number of times to convince themselves they were true. I was thrilled to hear that apparently on the questions to which they knew the answers, I was 100 per cent accurate. On those to which they themselves did not know the answer, my replies had seemed highly probable and, in many cases, later events had corroborated the dowsing reply. As a result, dowsing is now accepted and used as a legitimate addition to orthodox diagnostic techniques in their hospital and they also use it for selecting treatment and remedies.

It is fascinating how often information, unknown to a patient and indeed, at the time, to his orthodox advisers, will be discovered by dowsing. If a patient's doctor is interested, I can dowse for the various problems and then either apply healing and the various therapies we have developed, or refer the patient back to the doctor with notes on what I think is required, be it dietary change, manipulation by, for example, an osteopath, or some other form of treatment.

Because I have a particular interest in the nervous system, I find one of the most useful aspects of dowsing lies in assessing the well-being or otherwise of nerves throughout the body. This can be especially useful in the analysis of problems, as nerves do not show up on an X-ray picture. The maddening thing is that precisely *because* it is difficult to photograph nerves, my analyses cannot be easily verified, except circumstantially. I hope that current specialized research equipment will soon be available at a clinical level to provide this corroboration, or otherwise.

Like anyone else who has built up a theory on empirical evidence, I am prepared to accept that the rationale is open to correction in the light of research. It may be that it is not impediments in the nerve pathways that matter. The vital factor may perhaps be the bio-electrical operational system which interlocks physically with the nervous system, probably through the Schwann cells, the supportive structure of the neurones. Becker[2], amongst others, postulates that this system which transmits data using varying levels of direct current as its signal controls life functions such as the sensation of pain, tissue growth and healing. I am delighted that scientists are trying to find out more about the functions which control inadequate growth (such as arthritis), abnormal growth (such as, at the extreme end, cancer) and organic healing. Meanwhile, my unscientific concept of 'trapped nerves' provides a working hypothesis for finding and correcting trouble in the body, and dowsing is an invaluable aid in this.

Theories about Dowsing

All this may sound fairly strange and obviously I cannot demonstrate here that dowsing works. I shall try, however, to outline the possible explanations. None of them is as satisfactory as proving its efficacy for yourself.

Conscious and Subconscious

As we have said before, men and women are made up of a number of faculties as well as the physical body. One of the conscious aspects is the intellect and this faculty has been admired and cultivated in various cultures in the West for a number of centuries. We have ignored, as far as possible, the faculties of the subconscious and particularly of intuition which has been distrusted and even actively discouraged. The intuitive subconscious 'knows' a great deal more than we give it credit for. Our Western conditioning has been such that we find it extremely difficult to bring to our conscious notice things that are known by the subconscious. We have a highly effective 'filter' system between the subconscious and the intellect. This system, well known to the medical hypnotists under a different name, allows us to ignore information that does not seem to be relevant to our logically based view of the world and our part in it. Dowsing seems to be able to form a bridge for bringing to the conscious understanding of the intellect factors that are known in the subconscious. In the case of healing, the factors are probably known in the subconscious of both parties, but some mechanism is needed to reach them.

Hemispheres of the Brain

It might be helpful to look at this in terms of the structure of our perceptual mechanisms as we understand them. The cortex of the brain is subdivided into right and left hemispheres, and it has been maintained that the two sides have different functions. The left side is held to be responsible for such operations as logical thought, time-sequence analysis, categorizing and speech and is the dominant half wherein consciousness resides. The right hand side is concerned not with words and logic but with picture comprehension and maze solving and is capable of appreciating and synthesizing a complex whole. (In fact, the 'left brain' function is apparently not always physically situated on the left hand side, but as there are unquestionably two types of brain functioning it is convenient to label them 'left hemisphere-type function' and 'right hemisphere-type function'.)

When tested on a multi-channel electro-encephalograph, the majority of people show that most of the time they only use the left hemisphere of their brains. Maxwell Cade[3] and others consider that the integration of left and right-hemisphere functions in an uninhibited reciprocal transmission of nervous impulses across the corpus callosum (the great bridge of nervous tissue which unites the two halves of the brain) will, to a great extent, provide the union of conscious with unconscious mental activity. To my knowledge, little if any research has been done on dowsers, and it would be interesting to see if they would show symmetrical patterns. Other unusual abilities such as clairvoyance also give access to material unknown to the conscious mind. According to Cade, these abilities are certainly associated with changes in the encephalograph pattern towards a more bilaterally symmetrical and integrated form.

We are still left with the question: 'How does the subconscious know?' Once again, I cannot give a full answer but I put forward two potentially fruitful lines of investigation.

The Collective Unconscious

Jung[4] believed not only in the power and knowledge of the individual subconscious but in what he called the collective unconscious. From his endless observations and his own experiences he concluded that every individual subconscious can reach down and into the collective experiences and knowledge of mankind. Theoretically, our subconscious may be tapping the available knowledge in the collective unconscious and bringing it, via the dowsing bridge, to the notice of the conscious mind.

The Huna Code
The Kahunas,[5] the priesthood of an ancient religion in the Pacific, believed that every living thing can be linked, no matter what the distance, by a sort of mysterious thread, and they developed this in the so-called Huna Code. The subconscious could find out via this thread whatever it needed to know about the well-being or otherwise of any individual—or indeed of anything to which it was linked.

Attunement and Resonance
The Huna Code does not conflict with the concept that we mentioned earlier. If all matter is merely energy vibrating at a multitude of different rates, then it should be possible to pick up the various vibrations and tune in to them. Having tuned in, questions can be asked and replies received.

Mediumistic Possibilities
It is perfectly possible that dowsing may enable us to tune in not only to people, animals, plants and every other form of matter, but also to beings with every human attribute except a physical body, but I will leave this subject for consideration in the next chapter.

All that need concern us here is whether any of these hypotheses help us to make sense of what demonstrably works. If we are in touch through some level of our being, no matter what level, with everyone and everything on this planet then we can see a route by which we can ascertain well-being or otherwise.

Distant Dowsing and Absent Healing
In the popular mind, wave-lengths are associated with radio, television and telecommunications. These can work over quite phenomenal distances. The ability to pick up these wave-lengths depends, however, on the strength of the receiver. I think that dowsing is probably similar. It is relatively easy to tune in to local stations. In the same way, it is easier for many people to tune in to somebody or something that is physically present. Proximity is not vital, however, and I personally have always found distance irrelevant. Provided the set is powerful enough, or in other words provided the dowser can hold the concept of his subject adequately, distance makes no difference. I have already quoted the example of the doctors in Austria who found their questions satisfactorily answered by someone in Scotland.

I have not, unfortunately, taken part in any controlled scientific tests to verify (or otherwise) whether my long distance dowsing is accurate, and merely to quote individuals who claim that my analyses were subsequently corroborated is unsatisfactory. I would suggest that this is another legitimate area for research. It is probable that this capacity is similar to telepathy and experiments in this phenomenon conducted between Moscow and Leningrad and Moscow and Kerch have apparently been impressive enough to convince a number of scientific researchers in the U.S.S.R.[6] of its reality.

To push the radio analogy a little further, our sets (in other words ourselves) can act not only as receivers; they can also be used to transmit messages. Having tuned in, we can then actively resonate with the vibrations we pick up. We cannot prove this, but the simple concept of resonance is a familiar one to those who have studied any physics and, at its simplest, it means that by transmitting on the same wave-length we can reinforce and increase the strength of the original wave.

This, I suspect, is the basis for absent or distant healing, whereby the healer 'transmits' healing to an individual who may be many thousands of miles away. Some people feel it is important that the recipient should be asked in advance to try to 'tune in' at the same time but I have never found this necessary. Thousands of people are convinced that they received tremendous help from absent healing through a multitude of healers, but again little research has been done. Cade reports only one experiment. The well known healer Edgar Chase was seated in a room and instructed to commence absent healing on a patient in a separate room at a particular moment. The patient was unaware of the experiment but at the prearranged time, his brain wave pattern as measured on the multi-channel encephalograph (or 'mind mirror') changed to the unusual 'state five' which seems to be associated with healing. This suggests the reality of absent healing but is not in itself conclusive.

Surrogate Healing

It would seem to be helpful to have some sort of focus for the tuning-in process. I have tested a system of proxy or surrogate healing and have found it effective in a number of cases. Here, someone in good health is treated as the representative of a patient who, for a variety of reasons, cannot be touched. In my experience this has proved effective where the patient was suffering from a degenerative condition of the skeletal system which would have made any attempt to adjust or manipulate the defective areas totally unsuitable. In other cases, distance has been the problem. In a number of examples of both types the results have been very exciting and apparently successful. I use the word 'apparently' because in only one case was there a degree of corroboration from the medical authorities involved. In the others, the 'evidence' consisted of statements from the patients and relatives or close friends. I believe that the key factors include finding a proxy who is 'in resonance' at the critical frequencies with both the patient and the problem.

Radionics
Radionic instruments (familiarly referred to as 'the Box') also appear to work on the principle of resonance. In this case, equipment is used to enable the practitioner to tune in, diagnose and direct help. These instruments are obviously a great help to many people, but it is well known that the Box will work more effectively for some people than for others. My work with these instruments under the guidance of George and Marjorie Delawarr (who pioneered radionics in this country) and Roy Firebrace during the forties and early fifties convinced me that the box, like the pendulum, is an invaluable aid that amplifies signals available at a subconscious level but presents them in a more sophisticated form. It is, however, the practitioner that matters.

Funnily enough, practitioners in totally different fields are tentatively beginning to come to similar conclusions. One psychologist at the Royal Welsh Dental School, after years of working on the psychological aspect of dental pain, now says that he thinks that the procedure followed is less important than the person administering it from the psychometric point of view. I have already mentioned the work of Joe Navach. He has found through working with the N.A.S.A.-built instrument for measuring the Auricular Cardiac Reflex that some of those using the instrument can 'think' a positive Auricular Cardiac Reflex into the patient being measured. The results, even with this sophisticated machine, are therefore dependent on the practitioner.

Further Forms of Tuning In
You may find that after some practice, you barely need a pendulum. Some people find that they get a positive or negative 'feel' simply by rubbing their fingers together. I find that sometimes I can 'tune in' and get a hunch about somebody or something. This is perhaps the faculty for 'inspired guesswork'. I can double check the hunch by dowsing carefully with a pendulum which of course I always do when working with a patient or any other important project.

The Use of Dowsing in Different Fields
Dowsing is bringing into play something which is entirely natural, built into us from birth but not normally brought to the fore in our culture. It can be applied to any activity. I find it particularly useful for a number of things, including the selection of remedies and the

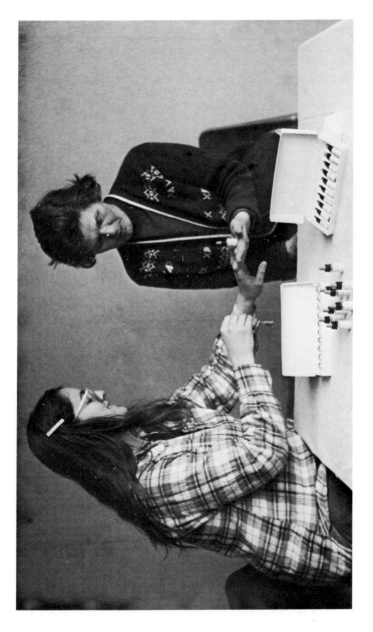

Figure 6. A member of the Westbank group dowsing for suitable remedies.

appropriate dosage. The British Society of Dowsers, however, lists successful dowsers whose particular interests include archaeology, finding old mines, repairing church bells and a multitude of other more everyday activities. Gardeners find it especially useful. If they wish to find out whether a particular plant will flourish in a given spot, they can either dowse to see whether the two are compatible or they can do their own soil analysis. It is much quicker to analyze soil by dowsing than by sending off samples to laboratories. The gardener merely holds a handful of soil in one hand and the pendulum in the other while running through a list of the appropriate minerals and whatever else gardeners like their soil to contain, finding out their presence or lack of them and ascertaining what, if anything, should be added to make a particular plant grow satisfactorily.

We are not all going to be brilliant dowsers in *every* field. I can use dowsing for healing but I am hopeless at finding lost articles. Others are extremely good at this but in turn may be no good at finding minerals. To use the analogy of the radio set just once more, we as the sets will find ourselves constructed to operate at maximum strength on some channels and less well on others. What we have to do is find our particular range of frequencies. This is one of the things that we are constantly helping people to do during our training sessions both at home in Scotland and on courses in various parts of this country and abroad.

Finding your own particular range is the first thing and the second is practice. Like any faculty that has lain dormant for many years, the dowsing ability will probably not be very active immediately. You have to work at it, gradually finding out your own code with whatever dowsing mechanism you may choose—and you must keep a very stern eye on the accuracy of your answers. Even now there are frequently times when I suspect that I am not tuning in properly and on these occasions I ask my wife, Patricia, to submit me to a test. Only if I am 100 per cent accurate will I return to the subject in hand. One cannot afford to make mistakes if someone's water supply, far less their health, is at stake!

Bibliography

1. Graves, Tom. *Dowsing: Techniques and Applications.* Turnstone Books, 1976.
   See also: Nielson, Greg and Polansky, Joseph. *Pendulum Power.* Exacalibur Books, 1981.
2. Becker, Robert O. Plenary lecture presented at the Second International Symposium on Bioelectrochemistry, Pont a Mousson, 1-5 October 1973. Published in *Bioelectrochemistry and Bioenergetics* 1974, pp 187-199.
3. Cade, C. Maxwell and Coxhead, Nona. *The Awakened Mind.* Wildwood House, 1980.

See also: Ornstein, Robert. *The Psychology of Consciousness.* Harcourt Brace, 1977.

Luria, A. R. The Working Brain. Penguin, 1973.

Beaumont, J. G. 'Handedness and hemisphere Function' in *Hemisphere Function in the Human Brain* edited by Diamond, S. J. and Beaumont, S. G. Halstead Press, New York, 1953.

4. Jung, Carl Gustav. *Collective Works.* Routledge and Kegan Paul, 1979.
5. Long, Max Freedom. *The Secret Science at Work.* De Vorss, California, 1953.
6. Gris, Henry and Dick William. *New Soviet Psychic Discoveries.* Sphere Books, 1980.

8. Extending Our Awareness

We have talked about tuning in and extending our awareness with particular reference to analyzing problems and helping people. The premise that we can do this opens up a much wider field of human potential. It is a field that is bedevilled by different terminologies and concepts as it embraces numerous approaches to man, his make-up and his relationship with the world in which he lives. Psychology, parapsychology, so called ESP, various religions and some schools of philosophy all attempt to explore and make sense of the demonstrable fact that man can and does have faculties which manifest themselves from time to time, but which we do not fully understand.

You may ask what place such topics have in a book about healing. I would answer that they are pertinent to man's realization of his full potential. As such, they come within my broader concept of healing as the process of becoming more whole and of sharing that increased well-being and understanding with others, including animals, plant life and the earth. Einstein put it extremely well when he said

> A human being is part of the whole, called by us 'Universe', a part limited in time and space. He experiences himself, his thoughts and feelings as something separated from the rest, a kind of optical delusion of his consciousness. This delusion is a kind of prison for us, restricting us to our personal desires and to affection for a few persons nearest to us. Our task must be to free ourselves from this prison by widening our circle of compassion to embrace all living creatures and the whole of nature in its beauty. Nobody is able to achieve this completely, but the striving for such achievement is, in itself, a part of the liberation and a foundation for inner security.

The Unsolicited Gift
Such a statement takes the pragmatic approach that the extension of our awareness through relaxation, meditation or a multitude of other techniques is essentially useful and leaves aside any consideration of ethical evaluation or of a spiritual aim. Mind, which interprets what we perceive with our senses, is obviously involved in any such

processes and mind is married to the activities of the brain. I like
Arthur Koestler's story [1] to illustrate what he calls 'the unsolicited gift'.

There was once an illiterate shopkeeper in an Arab bazaar, called Ali
who, not being very good at doing sums, was always cheated by his
customers—instead of cheating them, as it should be, So he prayed every
night to Allah for the present of an Abacus—that venerable contraption
for adding and subtracting by pushing beads along wires. But some
malicious djinn forwarded his prayers to the wrong branch of the
heavenly Mail Order Department, and so one morning, arriving at the
bazaar, Ali found his stall transformed into a multi-storey, steel-framed
building, having the latest IBM computer with instrument panels
covering all the walls, with thousands of fluorescent oscillators, dials,
magic eyes, etc; and an instruction book of several hundred
pages—which, being illiterate, he could not read. However, after days of
useless fiddling with this or that dial, he flew into a rage and started
kicking a shiny delicate panel. The shocks disturbed one of the machine's
millions of electronic circuits, and after a while Ali discovered to his
delight that if he kicked the panel, say three times and afterwards five
times, one of the dials showed the figure eight! He thanked Allah for
having sent him such a pretty abacus, and continued to use the machine to
add up to two and three—happily unaware that it was capable of deriving
Einstein's equations in a jiffy, or predicting the orbits of planets and stars
thousands of years ahead.

Ali's children, then his grandchildren inherited the machine and the
secret of kicking that same panel; but it took hundreds of generations
until they learned to use it even for the purpose of simple multiplication.
We ourselves are Ali's descendants—though we have discovered many
other ways of putting the machine to work, we have still only learned to
utilise a very small fraction of the potentials of its estimated hundred
thousand million circuits. For the unsolicited gift is of course the human
brain. As for the instruction book, it is lost—if it ever existed. Plato
maintains that it did once—but that is hearsay.

The potential of the computer is enormous and is not of itself good or
bad. The use to which it is put, however, is open to moral scrutiny. In
other words, the extension of our awareness and any abilities that may
follow in the wake of such an extension are neither good nor bad, but
like any human faculty, the way in which they are used can be
evaluated. The fact that any such extension tends to lead towards a
realization of some higher spiritual order, to religious experience, to a
sense of unity with an Absolute, or from the subconscious to some
'supraconscious' world I shall leave for another chapter—having, I
hope, indicated in this one sentence some of the difficulties of
terminology.

Extended Sensory Perception and Parapsychology
If we extend our awareness, consciously or unconsciously, we are also
extending that which we perceive with our senses. I would suggest that

healing and dowsing are only two aspects of man's natural ability to use his senses at a different level. For me, green-fingered gardeners, healers, dowsers, clairvoyants and exponents of every other form of special attunement are all using some aspect of the same ability, according to their own natural bent. They have not, in my view, got access to anything 'extra' which is why I use the phase 'extended sensory perception' in preference to the more common phrase 'extra sensory perception'.

Some aspects of what I would consider extended perception are taken for granted in our society and would not normally be considered as part of ESP. Green fingers are a case in point. I would include many artists and musicians who seem to perceive things in greater depth than the rest of us. They have, if you like, a more open path to the source of their inspiration; or, to put it another way, by using their senses at a different level they increase their creativity. Most other aspects of so-called ESP are often regarded variously with suspicion or derision. I suspect that behind this reaction frequently lurks a fear of phenomena that do not fit into our conditioned Western world picture. This fear can be seen even in relation to psychology which threatens to disinter disagreeable irrational depths and aspects of personality which the individual would rather not know about, and would certainly prefer not to share with others.

Psychology has, however, led the way in breaking down the old ideas of what maketh man. ESP, or parapsychology as it is now fashionable to name it, still has a long way to go, particularly in Britain, though there are signs that we are coming out of the 'ostrich phase'. The establishment in both the U.S.A. and U.S.S.R. have recognized that this area is worthy of attention, even if sometimes only for thoroughly materialistic reasons. Chairs of parapsychology have been set up in various universities, and finance has been made available to serious scientific researchers. This is unfortunately not yet the case in Britain where virtually all the work and research is still in the hands of enthusiastic individuals and a few independent societies.

The Filter System
A number of the experiments into the phenomena of ESP have illustrated very nicely the fact that everyone has the ability to sense things at a different level, but that their conscious mind refuses to accept what the subconscious perceives. I will only quote one such experiment because it is one that could easily be repeated by anyone wishing to verify the results. All that is required is to hire a few encephalographs.

In this experiment, a number of people were wired up to encephalographs, all of which had a time-recording device so that it was possible to know at what time any particular pattern was demonstrated. The subjects were put in different sound-proofed rooms and told to try and pick up a telepathic message sent out by an individual, himself kept under identical carefully controlled conditions. Only a very small percentage recorded the message correctly. The rest claimed that they could sense nothing. Every single encephalograph, however, registered a change in individual pattern at the time the 'message' was sent out and for the duration of it. This suggests that every subconscious registered the message, but that very few people could get the message past the filter and bring the material to the attention of the conscious mind.

As usual, I am not by any means the first person to think that our conscious brain 'filters' the input from the world around us. Aldous Huxley[2] quotes Bagson's theory that the function of the brain, nervous system and sense organs is in the main eliminative and not productive. Bagson apparently claimed that each individual is capable of remembering all that has ever happened to him and of perceiving everything that is happening everywhere in the universe. The brain's job is to protect us from being overwhelmed by this mass of knowledge, leaving only that tiny selection which is practically useful in so far that, as animals, our business is at all costs to survive. Huxley points out that, according to such a theory, each one of us is potentially Mind at Large, but to make biological survival possible, Mind at Large has to be filtered or, as he puts it, funnelled through the reducing valve of the brain and the nervous system. What comes out the other end, he says, is a measly trickle of the kind of consciousness which will help us to stay alive on the surface of this particular planet.

As Huxley also points out, the filter or reducing valve is reinforced by our gift (or is it a curse?) of speech. To formulate and express the contents of this 'measly trickle' of consciousness, man has invented and endlessly elaborated

> . . . those symbol-systems and implicit philosophies which we call languages. Every individual is at once the beneficiary and the victim of the linguistic tradition into which he or she has been born—the beneficiary in as much as language gives access to the accumulated records of other people's experience, the victim in so far as it confirms him in the belief that reduced awareness is the only awareness and as it bedevils his sense of reality, so that he is only too apt to take his concepts for data, his words for actual things . . . Most people most of the time know only what comes through the reducing valve and is consecrated as genuinely real by the local language.

Small wonder that we have difficulties in extending our awareness past the double barricade of filter or reducing valve and terminology! The physicists have long recognized the latter and expressed themselves in mathematical formulae.

Unblocking the Filter

We are potentially able to surmount these barricades as the filter can be bypassed or unblocked by accident or design. The former was very frequent in wartime as shock and fear are powerful 'blockbusters'. I suspect it was the trauma of seeing men appallingly wounded which opened a gateway for me and made me put my hands on them. Fear and danger can frequently call forth capabilities for clairvoyance and intuitive knowledge. On one occasion while manoeuvering at night in part of northern France which I had never previously visited, we came to a large house requisitioned for our use. It was far too close to the enemy to allow us to use any light. Standing in the hall, I found that I knew the layout of all the rooms in the house, their size, how many each would accommodate and where they were connected to each other. I gave precise orders accordingly. When the NCO returned having carried out my orders, he found it impossible to believe that I had no previous knowledge of the house as my description had been completely accurate.

I found myself aware of imminent danger in the nick of time on a number of occasions. In this I was not by any means alone and probably most people have heard of similar experiences in wartime — on both sides, of course, as God is not necessarily an Englishman!

As in the examples quoted, the spontaneous opening of the filter or reducing valve can obviously be extremely useful for the survival of the individual or of others. We can open the filter spontaneously and having discovered the possibilities we can then set about opening it at will. Healing as one of the manifestations of the widened filter can therefore start spontaneously but be consciously developed thereafter. The danger of opening up to the mass of available sensation and knowledge is that we may be overwhelmed if we cannot 'close down' again afterwards. Dowsing is one of the safest ways of penetrating the filter but other methods can accomplish similar results.

Relaxation exercises, meditation, hypnosis and a multitude of techniques developed by the various cultures and religions, using everything from drugs to dancing, all attempt to change our level of awareness. Some have a particular spiritual level in view, others are merely interested in extending their understanding with a view to helping ourselves and others. The positive benefits can be enormous.

Relaxation Techniques and Applied Meditation

I could not describe with authority all the various routes to the different levels of extended awareness, even if space permitted. Many of them can be deeply disturbing if carried out without knowledgeable instruction and help. The recent books by Carlos Castaneda[3] relating his experiences under the tuition of the Mexican Indian, Don Juan, for example, make this all too clear. Some people find they have to go into a trance state before the filter will relax its grip. Others can extend their awareness while retaining consciousness and control and it is this latter approach which we teach in our various courses.

Self Help

Physical relaxation techniques of various sorts are easy to learn and can take you as far as you wish to go. Few of us really relax properly in our daily lives, as putting your feet up and watching the T.V., reading a book or listening to a favourite record still leave numerous muscles taut. Contrary to general belief, we are rarely fully relaxed even in sleep. Effective relaxation involves gaining more awareness and then control of our bodies with the paradoxical intent of 'letting go' of them. As we consciously instruct every little muscle to relax, we can then 'listen' to what the various parts of our body can tell us through the subconscious, and we can become aware of tension or discomfort and slowly work on this in various ways. Our minds and our bodies can, in fact, learn to listen to each other and work in harmony, though it may take a great deal of practice to do this properly.

Some of the biofeedback instruments demonstrate the extent of the control that can be gained. For instance, someone working with thermocouples (instruments measuring body temperature) can learn to raise and lower their temperature at will, or even to lower the temperature of one hand and simultaneously raise the temperature of the other hand and to alternate the temperature of the hands on demand. Imagine the benefit of this sort of control for those with high blood pressure, for example. Very valuable work is in fact already being carried out in this field, both privately and under medical supervision in hospital. Numerous patients with high blood pressure and various heart complaints have been taught how to control their own problem without drugs. This has the obvious advantages of preventing both drug dependence and any adverse side-effects which so often can complicate medical treatment.

Admiral Shattock realized the power of the mind over the body and used it with very exciting but sometimes devastating results. Finding himself with serious medical problems which nearly always require major surgery, he discovered from the doctors everything he could about his illness. He then proceeded to issue some detailed instructions to his body on how to deal with the situation. The body obeyed him implicitly. Unfortunately, he left out a vital order, with the result that he very nearly died. His book[4], *Mind Your Body*, tells the story of his determined and ultimately successful efforts to restore his own health by what he calls 'contacting his autonomic mind' and it gives very practical instructions to those who would like to follow a similar course.

In short, complete control can be established and the intellect can override the subconscious for better or worse. Long experience, however, has persuaded me that very few people can achieve such a degree of discipline as Admiral Shattock. It is safer and simpler for most people to draw the attention of the subconscious to a problem and invite it to undertake the task of putting it right. This still calls for discipline, effort and persistence but the rewards can be dramatic and far-reaching. The Kahunas[5] taught this particular approach to problems and many of those in the West who recognize the interplay between physical tension, emotional stress and disease are now teaching various methods of affecting one's own health through the subconscious or 'autonomic mind'.

Creative Imagination and Symbols

Having established a working relationship with the body, or perhaps more properly with that part of the subconscious mind which controls the body, we can then introduce ourselves to other aspects and levels of the subconscious. I use the term subconscious very loosely to mean not only those levels of our own selves which are the study of psychologists, but also the unconscious factor unaffected by the rational filter which relates to the rest of existence. Those talking in terms of the individual subconscious talk about 'deeper' levels of consciousness. Those interested in ultimate reality (whatever that may be), rather than the everyday human concepts of reality, often talk in terms of 'higher states' of consciousness. Koestler[1] remarks that we may not be able to say what consciousness is but we can say whether there is more or less of it and also whether it is coarse or refined in texture.

Cade has taken this one step further as he claims to have established the existence of a measurable hierarchy of states of consciousness, each one a stage in a progressively more integrated pattern of electrical activity in the brain. It is a very difficult area to chart.

Once again, I come back to the practical point : exploring our consciousness helps us to identify and clear subconscious blocks and find and enhance our own creative talents. These may be in any field from mathematics to sculpture. They may be in the form of clairvoyance or healing or appear as the extension of any faculty; these talents may be less easily identified and show themselves as an ability to understand people and the world about us better. Maslow[6] distinguishes between two types of creativity in just this way. He noted that some people showed 'special talent' creativeness and that others showed what he called 'self-actualizing' creativeness. Such a capacity, says Maslow, is normal to most children but frequently lost in adulthood and shows itself as a tendency to do everything creatively, with a special kind of insight that has nothing to do with productivity or training.

'Creative imagination' can be a useful tool to explore the realms of what we loosely call the subconscious. By deliberately encouraging our capacity for fantasy, we allow a creative faculty to come out of hiding. What it produces may sometimes be illusion, but as we liberate and develop it we can 'tune in' through it to other knowledge known in the subconscious or the collective unconscious; we can thereby learn to discriminate the creative elements from the merely illusory.

At this point I should warn the reader that the potential for illusion will always be with us however experienced we may become, and the need for continuous monitoring by the intellect remains with us. No matter how wise we think we have become, we can always be tripped up! This highlights the value of comparing notes with a teacher or a group as the harmony between intellect and subconscious is difficult to achieve and maintain and we are not always our own best assessors.

Subconscious faculties do not necessarily express themselves in words. Once we start paying attention to them, we can begin to understand that some of the supposedly fanciful images produced are in fact useful signs and symbols that can impart information to us. We are already used to living with symbols in everyday existence. We need no words to tell us that the road ahead is twisting when we see a Z bend sign. We now have to learn about the symbols used by the subconscious. Volumes[7] have been written on the subject, but suffice it to say here that while there are undoubtedly some universal symbols, many of them are highly individual and it is potentially misleading to accept anyone else's interpretation of your symbols unless it 'feels' right to you.

Meeting People in Extended Consciousness

When deeply relaxed and in tune with another level of awareness, it is fairly common to see and talk to 'imaginary' people. They can appear very real and can, on occasions, be extremely helpful. 'They' could be a number of things apart from straight illusion. Some may be merely externalizations of aspects of oneself. Even so, discussion can be very useful. I find that on some occasions I see 'in my mind's eye' people whom I do not know. I feel as if they are physically present and I can describe them in great detail down to a mole on the cheek or a crooked thumb. Frequently I find that I have described a real person, very often someone who has asked for 'absent' healing.

Inner or Spirit Guides

Many people recognize that very personal helpers turn up to talk to them, assist with problems and generally guide them. You can, if you like, consider these 'guides' to be in reality a personalized form of one aspect of the subconscious. For personal reasons, I am sure that real 'people' who have every human attribute except a physical body are also around and prepared to help us.

Bibliography
1. Koestler, Arthur. *The Ghost in the Machine*. Hutchinson, 1976.
2. Huxley, Aldous. *The Doors of Perception*. Panther, 1977.
3. Casteneda, Carlos. *The Teachings of Don Juan*. Penguin, 1970.
4. Shattock, E. H. *Mind Your Body*. Turnstone Press, 1979.
5. Long, Max Freedom. *The Secret Science at Work*. De Vorss, California, 1953.
   Also see amongst many others:
   Assagioli, Roberto. *The Act of Will*. Wildwood House, 1974.
   Simonton, O. Carl, Matthews-Simonton, Stephanie and Creighton, James L. *Getting Well Again*. Bantam Books, 1980.
6. Maslow, A. H. 'The Creative Attitude' in *Explorations in Creativity* edited by Mooney, R. L. and Razik, T. A. Harper and Row, U.S.A., 1967.
7. Jung, Carl Gustav. *Man and His Symbols*. Pan Books, 1978.

9. The Discarnate World

It was in 1941 when I was temporarily back in Britain that I met Louisa Ashdown. She was a delightful, unpretentious woman with an unusual gift. She could sit in her drawing room chatting to her guests and simultaneously a voice, audible to everyone in the room, could be heard coming from a point anything up to ten feet away from her. While not denying the existence of ventriloquism, such a feat was totally impossible in the circumstances as the larynx cannot be used to produce two voices simultaneously. The evidence that I heard on numerous occasions was quite enough to convince me that the information imparted could not possibly be known to any of those present and the information was frequently expressed fluently in foreign languages of which Louisa Ashdown had no knowledge. One voice which addressed itself to me on many occasions showed a staggering knowledge of the French campaign in which I had recently been involved. I never discovered the identity of the speaker, but he was obviously a senior officer as he had far greater and wider knowledge of events than I could have from my lowly position of second lieutenant. His description of many critical situations in which I had been involved was graphic and detailed—and they were not subjects I had ever talked about except in the most general terms.

Until the end of 1942 and after the war I worked with a great many mediums or 'sensitives' as they are now known. In retrospect I realize how lucky I was to meet so many extraordinarily talented people. I could go on at length about the evidence that convinced me that survival after death is a reality regardless of one's religious concepts, but I will tell only one more story. It was in Edinburgh in 1949 that a group of people, myself included, was asked by the Psychic College in Herriot Row to test Helen Duncan. She had recently completed a term in prison for alleged fraudulent mediumship and it was felt that if she was to take up her work again, an independent test should be carried out.

The female members of the group stripped and searched her and then sewed her into a one-piece suit with no pockets or apertures, which covered her from elbow to knee. We sat in a room with enough light to read the small print in a diary. I know because I checked! In the space of ninety minutes, seventeen separate forms came into the room. Many of them materialized sufficiently to be touched and we all heard the individual voices, both male and female, which came from different points of the room and could not possibly have come from the medium's throat. This was evidence enough, but I was further surprised when one of the forms approached me. He thrust out two handless arms and said in Serbo-Croat, 'You'll remember that you buried me under the mimosa tree'. Nobody else in the room, far less Helen Duncan, knew any Serbo-Croat. I knew very little, but had picked up a smattering of the language and the dialects during the war when running a small sea-going unit, which included a number of Yugoslavs supplying military necessities to the Allied Forces in Yugoslavia. Certainly nobody else in the room with Helen Duncan could have known about the particular incident to which this related, but I remembered it well enough. Some Yugoslavs had been rescued and brought to Italy after some internal fighting and many of them had been severely mutilated. Some of them survived, but not by any means all and I remembered one who had had his hands brutally hacked off whom we buried under a mimosa tree.

The survival of death is a subject that Western man on the whole shies away from or denies hotly, even if he has not investigated the matter at all. Dr Johnson took a sensible view of the question; he remarked

> . . . that the dead are seen no more I will not undertake to maintain against the concurrent and varied testimonies of all ages and of all nations. There is no people, rude or learned, among whom apparitions of the dead are not related and believed. This opinion, which perhaps prevails as far as human nature is diffused, could become universal only by its truth: those that never heard of one another would not have agreed in a tale which nothing but experience could render credible. That it is doubted by single cavillers can very little weaken the general evidence; and some who deny it with their tongues confess it by their fears.

There is of course a great deal of well attested evidence for survival for anyone who does not wish to take my word for it. As an example, Eileen Garrett, one of Britain's outstanding mediums with whom I shared many fascinating sessions, worked in America in the 1940s and submitted herself to rigorous tests under scientific conditions. The results of these tests were some of the factors that convinced many scientists that they should pay more attention to parapsychology, a subject that is now accepted at a number of universities in the United States. The evidence for Eileen Garrett's abilities and those of numerous other gifted individuals is available through the libraries of the Society for Psychic Research and the College of Psychic Studies. More recently, doctors began to study patients who had clinically 'died' and then been resuscitated. Their conclusions were that consciousness seemed to continue after death[1].

Teaching and Help from the Discarnate

I have not brought up the subject of the survival of death purely for its own sake. All the phenomena associated with mediumship is interesting and of value in that it alerts us to the reality of the Christian message of life after death. The main point, however, is that we can obtain enormous help from the discarnate (who include not just the so-called dead but other beings who may never have been incarnate), and I cannot stress too strongly that I feel it is both stupid and ungrateful to ignore it. It is equally stupid, of course, to suspend our critical faculties when communicating in this as in any field. I can only say that I (and I am not alone) am immensely grateful for the help and advice I have received over the years. This has included advice on my own health and a tremendous amount of information on how to help others. It sometimes takes the form of detailed diagnosis of individual patients or selection of remedies or suggestions of other possible sources of help.

Healing has been known in all parts of the world throughout the ages, and in every era many practitioners have given credit to some 'spiritual' source of help. This is true of the ancient Chinese, Egyptians and Greeks, of the Indian traditions, of Shamanism[2] as it was (and in some cases still is) practised in parts of Africa, Asia, Australia and the Americas. It is true of a great number, though not all, of the healers in the Western world. The difficulty lies in the definition of 'spiritual'. Do we mean that we can receive help from some greater spiritual or divine order with an inherent value system, or do we mean help from 'spirits', including the dead? I maintain that both are possible but Western cultures find it particularly difficult to accept the latter. Thus, healers who claim that they have spiritual 'guides' are often regarded as a little strange. Others claim that they are channels for divine assistance or that they recognize a 'life force' and give it different names such as *prana* or *mana* and attribute slightly different characteristics to it. The internal controversies can be bitter, but perhaps it is at least a start if man recognizes an unknown factor. Leaving aside for the moment any considerations of a greater spiritual order, I maintain that part of the so-called spiritual world is already within our grasp and demonstrably part of our lives.

Summary of Objections

There are many who will say that any notion of contact with a spiritual or discarnate world is unscientific and therefore impossible. From my point of view, spiritual help is an enormous asset, but I must stress again that extended sensory perception, including healing, works regardless of any belief or lack of it and, as experiments show, would seem to be subject to 'natural', if as yet incompletely understood laws. Do we perhaps dub 'supernatural' that which is in fact 'natural'? At any rate, many rational Westerners study or even practise healing without any reference to spiritual or discarnate elements.

I know that many people would like to think that contact with the discarnate world is impossible nonsense because if it is not, all sorts of alarming spectres arise. 'Messing about with spirits', many say, is either dangerous or wrong or both. While I admit that dealing with the discarnate has its dangers, I cannot accept that it is *ipso facto* wrong. To say that communication with the discarnate and spiritual worlds is *always* morally wrong because *sometimes* it can be dangerous and *sometimes* it is misleading is illogical. It would seem to me that because there are dangers we must learn more about it so that we can discriminate, sifting the valuable and the helpful from the destructive and misleading and, of course, the fraudulent.

Many of those in the West who say that contact with a spiritual world is wrong base their arguments on the teachings of the Christian church. The church's arguments are many and varied but broadly speaking they can be summarized as variations on two themes.

Firstly, they would claim that any genuine as opposed to fraudulent spiritual communication that does not come directly from God must be or is probably from the Devil. I submit, for reasons which I will put forward in a moment, that this judgement was reached for practical and political rather than ethical considerations. Secondly, they claim that whether the level of information imparted from supposedly spiritual sources is valued as good, bad or indifferent, the very excitement of communicating with discarnate sources can distract man from his proper task of aspiring to follow the Divine Will. There is some truth in both arguments in that the spiritual level or value of mediumistic information is immensely variable. A great deal of popular interest in séances is purely sensational and, instead of regarding contact with a spiritual world with reverence and a genuine desire to attain understanding and wisdom, some mediumistic contact can be debased to mere 'spirit bothering'.

The assessment of the value of any communication is of paramount importance. The question is surely that of authority. Who is going to be the judge and controller? Should any organization have a permanent monopoly and a blanket power of veto? This issue is not limited to Christianity. It is a universal problem, similar to that of parents throughout the world who have to consider when, if ever, they should allow their children to make their own judgements.

The Christian Background to Contact with Spirits

If you look up St Paul's first letter to the Corinthians, you will find an excellent dissertation in chapters twelve to fourteen on the various aspects of extended sensory perception, including mediumship, which Paul called the gifts of the spirit. He encouraged his listeners to practise these gifts. He made the vital point (first letter to the Thessalonians, Chapter 5) that we should test the spirits and sometimes reject them as in the case quoted in the Acts of the Apostles, Chapter 16. He *never* said ignore them. St John's first general epistle also makes the assumption that we will contact spirits through prophets or mediums and tells us not to believe *every* spirit, but to try them to see whether they are of God. Mediumship through the so-called oracles or prophets played a regular part in the early church, notably in the Church at Corinth founded by St Paul. The first great Latin father of the church, Tertullian, who lived in Carthage (circa 155-225) gave a fascinating description of mediumship in his essay 'On the Soul'.[3]

> We have amongst us a sister whose lot it has been to be favoured with gifts of revelation, which she experiences in the Spirit by ecstatic vision amongst the sacred rites of the Lord's Day in the Church; she converses with angels and sometimes even with the Lord; she both sees and hears mysterious communications; some men's hearts she discerns and she obtains directions for healing for such as need them. . . After the people are dismissed at the conclusion of the sacred services, she is in the regular habit of reporting to us whatever things she may have seen in vision; for all her communications are examined with the most scrupulous care, in order that their truth may be probed. 'Amongst other things' she says, 'there was shown to me a soul in bodily shape and a spirit appeared to me; not, however, a void and empty illusion, but such as would offer itself to be even grasped by the hand, clear and transparent and of an ethereal colour, and in form resembling that of a human being in every respect'. This was her vision and for her witness there was God, and the apostle is a fitting surety that there were to be Spiritual Gifts in the church.

Here we have spiritual help with healing, direct contact with God, with a hierarchy of spiritual beings (angels?) and with other souls or spirits.

It is of particular interest that the early church had no objection to the 'oracles' contacting intermediary spirits rather than demanding direct communication with God Himself all the time. If we accept a hierarchy, including the communion of saints, contact need not be with God Himself. It is of course vital to keep all our powers of judgement on the alert, but I find it very sad that for so many centuries we have been led to believe that if any communication does not come straight from God, it must automatically be from the Devil. The acceptance of a hierarchy of beings including 'dead' human beings (the communion of saints?) has to me always made perfect sense. As a soldier I frequently had to accept an order from a senior officer, even if it was delivered by a junior. I did not demand to see Montgomery himself before I carried them out, although on many occasions I would require specific corroboration before taking action. In the same way, we are encouraged in the New Testament to test any would-be spiritual guide by demanding proof of authenticity and motive. As in the case quoted by Tertullian the communications must be examined with most scrupulous care.

If mediumship was a valued part of the early church, why is it in such ill repute with the authorities today? If we are to test the spirits (but not ignore them) and see they be of God, then surely the men of God should be able to help and guide us in the matter. The established churches, however, are very unhappy about spiritualism. They are of course correct in assuming that if there are 'good' spirits there are probably also 'bad' ones, but they seem to have used this as the reason for pushing the whole subject under the carpet and banning it if possible. The basis of this probably lies once more in the politics of early church history.

The scholars dispute whether the passage in Tertullian concerning the medium refers to a Catholic or a Montanist service. The Montanists, as you may remember, were a group of Christians in Phrygia noted for their healers and what we would now call mediums, particularly Montanus himself and two women called Prisca and Maximillia. Their influence spread far afield and impressed many of the leading Christians, including Tertullian himself. The fact that there is a dispute about whether this service was influenced by Montanism or not implies that other churches, too, had their mediums; this is confirmed by the frequent references to 'oracles' or 'prophets' in the various Church Orders, of which the Didache, already quoted, is the first known example. The church, while accepting both healers and oracles, made it quite clear that the spirits had to be evaluated to see if they were 'of God'. If it was satisfactorily ascertained that this was the case, the oracles were much revered. The Montanists were therefore not really out of step, except in that the leaders were obtaining considerable influence which was a threat to the other arm of authority, the priesthood. Tertullian claims that the Bishop of Rome had already sent letters aimed at placating the troubles in Phrygia and recognizing the Montanists as orthodox, but at the persuasion of Praxeus and his lobby these letters were recalled. Having been within an inch of acceptance, the Montanists were then branded as heretics and excommunicated.

The priesthood over the ensuing years managed to gain the ascendance and in time were left unchallenged. The 'oracles of God' disappeared and any lay person demonstrating their gifts was promptly stigmatized as a servant of the Devil. Tertullian could well say of Praxeus that 'He drove out prophecy and brought in heresy and he put the Comforter to flight.' It seems that Montanus did become something of a spiritual megalomaniac, but the baby was thrown out with the bath water, so to speak, when disapproval of Montanus led to a ban on prophecy or mediumship.

The churches have cut themselves off from regular contact with the spiritual world through lay mediums ever since. It was not until the nineteenth century when the spiritualist movement started that the subject was opened up once more. The church authorities found themselves in a position equivalent to that of a government which, for many generations, has successfully upheld prohibition. When certain of the population rediscover alcohol, there is no one who fully understands its effects on man or who can discriminate between the respective values of crude alcohol and vintage claret. If the ban on alcohol is lifted, many of the least wise may become addicted to the cheapest and most damaging forms of neat alcohol, and this seems to corroborate the wisdom of prohibition. If, however, an essential part of the government's ancient constitution can be shown to advocate the discriminating use of alcohol, then the government must surely try to rediscover the old skills of production and help to guide the population towards a wise appreciation of them—while pointing out the dangers of licentious use of some undoubtedly damaging forms of drink.

The church's attitude is in many ways understandable but unfortunate in that is has cut us off from so much help. The Catholics regard the whole subject of contact with the 'realm of shades' as too dangerous for the lay population, though opinion on diabolic influence varies amongst the authoritative writers and there are some who think communication with spirits useful[4]. The Protestant churches on the whole find it more difficult than the Catholics even to accept the possibility of communication. Archbishop Lang and Archbishop Temple appointed a committee to investigate spiritualism in 1937. The committee took over two years to prepare their report and in fact did not come to a unanimous conclusion. The majority report was signed by seven out of the ten members. The House of Bishops then pigeon-holed the report for some nine years, when somehow or other it was leaked to the press. The conclusions reached by a Church of England Committee of course cannot be representative of the views of all its own authorities, far less those of any other church, but it is so well expressed that it is worth quoting.

The seven signatories of the Majority Report[5] came to the conclusion that

> . . . certain outstanding psychic experiences of individuals, including certain experiences with mediums, make a strong *prima facie* case for survival and for the possibility of spirit communications while philosophical, ethical and religious considerations may be held to weigh heavily on the same side.

They thought that 'it is probable that the hypotheses that they (communications through mediums) proceed in some cases from discarnate spirits is the true one'. They concluded that 'in general we need much more freedom in our recognition of the living unity of the whole church, in this world and in that which lies beyond death' and that spiritualism, if used with care and due recognition of the pitfalls, can fill up 'the gaps in our knowledge so that where we already walked by faith, we may now have some measure of sight as well'.

As the report states, it is more than worrying if people allow 'an interest in spiritualism, at a low level of spiritual value, to replace that deeper religion which rests fundamentally upon the right relation of the soul to God himself'. On the other hand, the report admits that 'if spiritualism does, in fact, make such an appeal to some, it is at least in part because the church has not proclaimed and practised its faith with sufficient conviction'. In addition, they make it clear that the recognition of discarnate concern for us 'cannot do otherwise . . . than add a new immediacy and richness to (our) belief in the Communion of Saints'. They add that 'There seems to be no reason at all why the Church should regard this vital and personal enrichment of one of her central doctrines with disfavour', so long as it does not distract Christians from their contact with God.

The report therefore regards spiritualism as both real and useful but the signatories make the vital point that we (and in this they include the lay population as well as the authorities) must use our powers of spiritual apprehension as fully and honestly as possible.

> It is true [the report admits] that there are quite clear parallels between the miraculous events recorded in the Gospels and modern phenomena attested by spiritualists. And if we assert that the latter must be doubted because they have not yet proved capable of scientific statement and verification, we must add that the miracles, and the Resurrection itself, are not capable of such verification either.

The report goes on to say that Christians accept the Gospels not because of the wonders but because they . . . 'ring true to the deepest powers of spiritual apprehension. *But if this is so, we must clearly apply the same criteria to the claims of spiritualists*' (my italics). In other words, we *can* have 'deep powers of spiritual apprehension' and these, together with our intellectual powers of reason, must be rigorously applied when dealing with mediumistic communications.

The Dangers: Spirits and Mediums Good and Bad
The report stresses the dangers and the possibilities for distortion and delusion. Just being dead is not going to make anyone particularly different, so I quite agree that there are going to be those who are malicious or downright destructive as well as the wise, kindly, stupid

and indifferent. We are quite accustomed to this in our normal lives. The odd politician, accountant, doctor, lawyer, and cleric has been discovered to be a crook but that does not mean that we ban politics, accountancy, the medical or legal professions and the clergy. We have to use our discrimination and, when necessary, ask for references. On every occasion I have found that those discarnate beings who make it their business to assist are prepared to take a great deal of time and trouble to establish their authenticity by, for example, showing a knowledge of intensely personal matters and I think this 'testing' is extremely important. Above all, we have to use our spiritual and moral understanding before committing ourselves.

As with the dead, so with the living. There are many brilliant mediums, but I am the first to admit that this whole field (like healing) is particularly open to abuse and fraudulence. This highlights the need for finding out more about it so that we can distinguish the good from the bad. Even the very best medium will of course have an 'off day'. Some of the most celebrated violinists occasionally play flat! And even in a trance state, it is frequently difficult for the medium to withdraw his or her personality sufficiently and this may inadvertently colour the message.

Do-It-Yourself Mediumship

It has been marvellous to have had the chance to experience the gifts of so many brilliant mediums. We can, however, if we are lucky, do the job to a certain extent for ourselves. If you like, it is similar to installing one's own telephone at home rather than going to the post office every time one wants to make a call. The telephone may not always work to order and it is possible to get a faulty line—and this can be true whether at home or in the post office.

I first discovered that my own capacity for direct mediumship was a reality when I was asked to give a talk to a large audience in Edinburgh in 1949. I was to share a platform with Helen Hughes, a famous medium, and had, with considerable trepidation, prepared a speech at short notice as I was merely a substitute for a very eminent speaker who had fallen ill. Subsequently I was told by Helen Hughes and three other clairvoyants in the audience that they had 'seen' a discarnate being step onto the platform with me. He had allowed me to start my talk and then stepped forward and placed a hand between my shoulder blades, whereupon I folded my notes, spoke for the allotted 45 minutes and sat down. The talk was well received but it bore no relation to my carefully prepared script! This has happened to me so frequently since that I can no longer be surprised, though I sometimes listen with interest to tape recordings of what I have said as I hear myself talking about matters that I did not think I knew. This can leave me at a loss when asked to authenticate my statements!

Sometimes I realize that I am 'off beam' and have to make corrections. One learns to recognize this with practice. If we go back to the analogy of the telephone, crossed or faulty lines are an occupational hazard of communicating. So do not assume that by dialling the White House, your information comes straight from the President; you may have got a crossed line to a small boy in Birmingham. Let him supply evidence of who he is, and keep your powers of judgement sharp for evaluating the worth of the information. In the last resort we have free will, and it is perfectly possible to ignore instructions if they seem likely to cause more harm than good.

Out of the Body Activity
Incidentally, we are all quite capable of operating without our bodies whether we are alive or dead. Louisa Ashdown was extremely perturbed when she 'saw' and spoke to me in London in 1943 even though I was physically many hundreds of miles away. She put down what I told her in her diary and, knowing that in reality I was fighting in North Africa, she wondered whether she should tell my mother I was dead. Luckily, she didn't. When I returned to England, she showed me her diary. There was my account of a small but particularly unpleasant incident in Tunisia, in which I had once again very nearly been killed—but not quite!

There was a small girl in Perthshire whom I knew purely on account of my spare-time hobby which was teaching show jumping to members of the Pony Club. She fell ill and as she was not responding to treatment, her mother (whom I did not really know at all) rang up a mutual friend to see if I would be prepared to help. Unfortunately, I was away and could not be contacted. The friend, having talked to me about telepathy in the past, endeavoured to send me a telepathic message stressing the severity of the child's illness. The rest of the story came from the child. She was sitting up in bed the next morning, her fever symptoms gone and loudly demanding breakfast. Her mother expressed surprise and delight. 'Don't be silly, mummy', came the response. 'You know that the man from the Pony Club, Major MacManaway, came to see me last night.' Her mother looked blank. 'Yes, he held his hands over my tummy and it was very hot and then he told me I'd be all right in the morning. And I am.'

Whether you call it astral travel or any other high-sounding name, this ability has been known in many parts of the world for centuries. Brian Inglis, in his book *Natural and Supernatural*[6] quotes many stories of confounded European travellers who found that the wise men in parts of Africa and elsewhere could slip into a trance and 'go' many miles and back in a night, bringing with them physical evidence and subsequently corroborated news as proof of their journey.

We really are more than just physical beings. We can operate without our bodies and we can do our best to help or hinder mankind, whether we are alive or dead.

Bibliography
1. Moody, Raymond. *Life After Life.* Corgi, 1977.
2. Halifax, Joan. *Shamanic Voices.* Penguin, 1980.
3. Tertullian, 'De Anima 9'. Ante-Nicene Christian Library quoted in *A New Eusebius. Documents illustrative of the History of the Church to A.D. 337.* SPCK, 1957.
4. For a selection of both sides of the Catholic argument, see the following:
   Crehan, Joseph. *Spiritualism.* The Incorporated Catholic Truth Society, 1979.
   Gatterer, Fr. Alois. 'Der Wissenschaftliche Okkultismus' 1927.
   Roure, L. 'L'Eglise Catholique et le Spiritisme' in essay on 'Spiritsme' in Dic. Theol. Cath. XIV 15-7-2522, 1940.
5. *The Church of England and Spiritualism.* Psychic Press (no date).
6. Inglis, Brian. *Natural and Supernatural.* Hodder and Stoughton, 1978.

10. Development of the Healing Ability

We frequently talk of the work of a musician, a poet or a lecturer as 'inspired'. What exactly do we mean? Sometimes, the source of inspiration is obvious. The passion of a love-affair, whether it brings agony or ecstasy, often calls forth from an artist some of his greatest work. This to me can be explained in terms of the transformation of enormous sexual and emotional energy (the sacral and heart chakras) into artistic expression. But sometimes there is no obvious source of inspiration, and yet we recognize, as in the case of the young Mozart, that someone can produce inspired work. Inspiration by what or by whom? I maintain that, in many cases, work that we recognize as beyond the normal capabilities of a child or of a person who we know to be talented, but not always exceptional, is really the result of unrecognized mediumship. The inspiration may be divine or it may be satanic. Some may have a 'hot line' to God or the Holy Spirit, others may have to make do with an emissary. Both the ability to transform our own energies into other creative areas and the ability to receive inspiration can be developed.

Natural and Supernatural
We talk of people being inspired by love, by nature, by the mountains and the trees. We talk of divine and spiritual inspiration. To me, the divisions between natural and supernatural are man-made and artificial: it is merely that our Western cultures understand the one but not the other. The increasing knowledge made available by science is amending the boundaries between 'natural' and 'supernatural' and I am not alone in believing that one day the laws of nature will be seen to embrace not only what we currently conceive as 'natural law' but also what we sometimes call 'divine ordinance'. If all matter is energy vibrating at an infinite number of wave-lengths, we can 'tune in' and resonate. However, we are more than 'matter'; we are not just our physical bodies, and we can communicate without our bodies. This, I maintain, is a natural ability, though the West does not recognize it as

such. Furthermore, if our bodies are not necessary, and we can communicate with those who no longer have a body, we merely have to recognize an additional factor, more 'people' in fact, when we extend our natural ability to tune into the earth and all the more obvious forms of life we sense around us.

If we start thinking in terms of God, or a Universal Intelligence or some such concept, then perhaps we can talk of the supernatural. But part of the so-called spiritual world is already within our grasp and, I think, demonstrably part of our lives. For this reason, I maintain that our current divisions between the natural and supernatural are incorrect. There is probably no deep divide between the natural or supernatural, but rather they are a continuum with discarnate humans forming a link between our incarnate consciousness and the workings of some greater spiritual consciousness. We can leave the idea of a greater spiritual world out of our calculations if we wish, (though I find this impossible myself) but we ignore the discarnate world to our own disadvantage. For the bulk of Western society to continue to do so without any attempt at investigation is for me extraordinarily out of keeping with the supposedly fearless twentieth century spirit of open-minded scientific enquiry.

Is Belief Necessary?
I am not asking anyone to believe what I say. Nearly everyone who comes to our centre does so as a last resort because they are ill and are not responding to orthodox therapies. They do not necessarily believe in anything at all and I do not ask them to do so. Healing, like all the other faculties mentioned, works regardless of belief and I think that personal experience is infinitely more valuable than theory. I have always had a very soft spot for the apostle Thomas who refused to believe until he had seen the risen Jesus for himself and felt the wounds with his own hands. The important thing was that Thomas was prepared to go and have a look and he did not angrily shrug off the whole story as nonsense unworthy of his attention. Just as important is the fact that the Master was prepared to offer such proof. He allowed Thomas to touch Him and to place his hands in the wound in His side. I am sure that we can still ask for 'proof'. Even if faith is eminently desirable, it is mentioned specifically by St Paul as a 'gift' and if something is a gift, then some may not possess it.

Very frequently, people who have come to see us because they wish to be rid of pain and illness become intrigued when they find that healing, irrational though it may seem, has helped them. They start to ask questions. I can try to answer them but then I can suggest that it might be more interesting to test my theories for themselves rather than to rely on talk or books. They can then come to any of the courses which we run in Scotland and elsewhere to find out firstly whether they can help themselves and secondly to see whether there is any reality in my talk of extended awareness and the value of the shared experience.

Discerning and Developing Latent Gifts

By learning to relax and listen, both to our bodies and to our inner selves, we start to discern our own creative talents. Perhaps it would be more accurate to say that, given a chance, they bubble to the surface. Once the gifts have been recognized, they can be developed and applied.

I find the analogy of musical talent a useful one. A child may naturally express a love and aptitude for music and it is then up to the teacher to bring out that gift and teach the skills of musical expression. Child and teacher between them should explore the possibilities of expression so that he or she can apply both gift and skill to singing or composition or playing a musical instrument. Many a child is not obviously musical, however, and in this case it is up to the teacher to recognize the latent ability. This happens in numerous schools throughout the country where, for example, all children are tested to see if they can join the choir, should they wish to do so. It is not just those who clamour to join who are included.

In any creative expression, both a gift and skill are involved. Once the gift is recognized, it is possible to develop it in a number of ways and people can learn to transform their own energy for use at the creative outlet. What the composer inspired by love is doing spontaneously can be consciously brought about. Finding a dearth of educational facilities after the last war, my wife and I founded a centre in our small family home in Scotland with the specific aim of helping not only those who request healing but also those who wish to discover, develop and apply their own gifts.

The Power of the Group

For this kind of development, it is enormously helpful to work with a harmonious group rather than by oneself. It would seem that the amount of energy available to all the individuals in a group is greater than the sum of the component parts. We are already well aware of this phenomenon in its negative manifestations as seen in the Nazi rallies or even some of today's football crowds. In its positive expression it can be equally powerful, and a group of people working together in harmony with each other and with their project seems to transform energy in a particularly effective way.

I find the power of a group particularly useful when working on some problem, more often than not for me the problem of a patient who is not responding fully to my treatment. Times out of number, through asking for the help of a group, the problem is sorted out. The power of a group is useful both when extending our awareness through

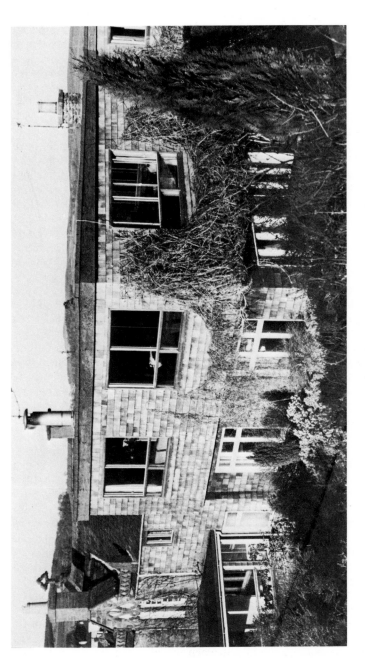

Figure 7. Westbank has grown over the years. The original cottage can be seen on the left.

applied meditation and when specifically trying to help others. Maxwell Cade has tested the theory in practical, physical terms by looking at the effects on the electrical activity of the brain when five or six healers work together in treating a patient. As each of the healers joins the team, the amplitude of the patient's 'fifth state' pattern (the pattern that seems to be associated with healing) increases.

Applying Extended Awareness in Daily Life
The contemplatives undoubtedly play a vital and very real part in maintaining and increasing the well-being of our world, but for most of us in the West, life consists of doing things. The talents we can discern and the channels to our inspiration that open up can be put into everyday practice and I am not in any way suggesting that everyone has to meditate all day. On the contrary, I am merely stating that extending our awareness enhances rather than hinders our normal life. The object of the exercise is to enhance the quality of our own lives, and then to share that well-being with our neighbours and environment. This, to me, comes within the concept of healing and 'making more whole'.

The possibilities are as many as there are individuals. By adding greater understanding and inspiration, people will dance better or play football better or cook better or design houses better. They can 'do their own thing' but improve upon it and by so doing enhance the quality of life for others.

Sometimes we can help those who wish to develop a specific latent gift. For example, those who wish to develop their healing or dowsing ability in certain fields may either train with us or be guided elsewhere.

The Feminine Attributes
I cannot leave the subject of developing human potential without bringing in another angle. In the broadest terms, what we have been talking about could be described as intuition. This is an attribute that has always been thought of as feminine. This does not mean that it is the sole prerogative of women. I like the Jungian concept that each of us, whether male or female, bears within us the attributes of the opposite sex. We know that this is true physiologically in that we all bear the prototype of both sexual attributes (although only one side will develop). It is also true psychologically, so that, as we all know, a woman can have all the intellectual and analytical qualities which are sometimes thought to be 'masculine' traits and a man can be as intuitive as a woman. Indeed, to operate fully, we all need to develop both sides of our natures. Irene Claremont de Castillejo [1] puts it very clearly when she explains that a woman's mind, although it can operate perfectly well with the 'focused consciousness' of a man, frequently operates at a level of 'diffuse awareness'. At this diffuse level she has an

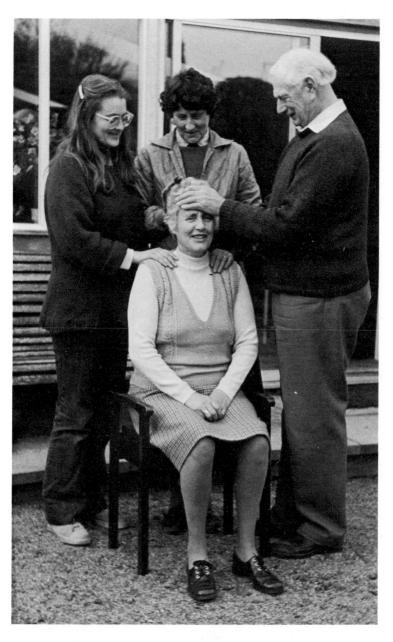

Figure 8. Treating a patient with help from a small group.

understanding and power far beyond the usual range of a man (unless he makes the effort to develop his 'feminine' side), and she is here in closest harmony with her deep feminine self, with nature and with those who surround her.

The trouble is that for many centuries in our Western culture, man has glorified his intellectual, rational side and poured scorn on the feminine aspects of 'irrational' intuition. He has even brain-washed women to believe that he is right though, luckily, he has not been able to kill the attributes themselves. Whenever I am lecturing, I am well aware of the fact that very few of the women present are giving me their full attention. They are listening hard and intelligently, but they are capable of thinking of a number of things at once. A woman can be writing a letter, keeping an eye on the stew, and subconsciously listening for the baby's cries (which she will hear, incidentally, despite the hubbub of radio, television or talk which drowns them for everyone else) all at the same time.

Despite this patent ability to operate at a diffuse level, women have been taught to be ashamed of this vital part of their nature. When they sometimes startle men by their perception or some inspired (that word again!) guess, they tend to look blank when questioned and then slightly shamefaced. 'Oh it was just intuition or something', *Just* intuition?!

As in the inner world, so in the outer. It is not coincidence that women have, on the whole, been denied any real part in the running of our society in the West until very recent years. This is an enormous subject and I can only touch on the history of the male-female struggle, which could perhaps be seen as intellectual suspicion of intuition. I like the concept expressed at one point in the Egyptian tradition when the Pharaoh was purportedly two people at once, one man and one woman. Only when both were present could anything important be done. Man expresses his everyday existence in his symbols and his gods. The Judaic tradition adheres to the idea of a father God and this continues in the Christian teaching. The Virgin Mary filled the gap, but even she has been given a pretty turbulent reception through the centuries, denigrated at the peak of Protestant zeal as the 'whore of Rome'. It is of interest that, although they have not yet been ratified by the Vatican as 'genuine', there has been a great spate of visions of the Virgin Mary in Europe in the last half century.[2] I would suggest that this is indicative of mankind's need for recognition of the feminine principal.

Women are at last beginning to take their place alongside men, though not without a struggle. At the moment, the competitive element is inevitably running high. Gradually, I hope the mutual suspicions will subside and woman, who is currently and rightly proving that her intellect can be as good as any man's, will also bring to full recognition her 'diffuse awareness', so that the two great instruments for understanding our world, intellect and intuition, can work together.

Bibliography
1. de Castillejo, Irene Claremont. *Knowing Woman: A Feminine Psychology.* C. G. Jung Foundation for Analytical Psychology, Hodder and Stoughton, 1973.
2. Chevallier, Bernard and Goulez, Bernard. *Je vous salue Marie.* Fayard, Paris, 1981.

11. Environmental Factors in Health and Healing

Whatever you like doing, and especially whatever you like eating or drinking, there is bound to be someone who will tell you it is bad for you. Before I go any further, I would like to stress that I am not advocating that we radically change our ways of life overnight, opt out of the stresses of modern society, ignore modern technology and turn into fasting ascetics. Man is incredibly resilient, both in body and mind, but he is perpetually bombarded by factors within his environment which are potentially damaging. Some he may shrug off (though another individual may be unable to do so), others he succumbs to. The difficulty is recognizing the particular factor that is harming an individual. This has now become one of the permanent specialities at our Centre where, by asking questions and dowsing, we are able to identify the trouble makers.

Some people can smoke all their lives without any noticeable ill effects. Should you contract lung cancer, however, you are probably not helping medical treatment if you continue to smoke sixty cigarettes a day and you cannot blame the doctors if treatment is not successful. We have to take some responsibility, both as individuals and as a society, for our health. This means being aware of the potential dangers, whether they be self-induced (smoking, overeating, over-work, etc.) or part of the external environment, widespread pollution being probably the most obvious factor. This includes everything from the recognized dangers of the lead content of petrol or radioactive fall-out to the more controversial side effects of much technological progress. It also means being aware of *yourself*, of your own psyche and your own 'soma' (body). It means listening to any warnings that your own particular system is running into trouble—and doing something about it. You cannot expect a doctor, therapist or a healer to put you right permanently if you go straight back and repeat whatever it was that made you ill in the first place or, more subtly, if you deny all responsibility for your own illness. It is arguably bad luck that you caught mumps, but are you running your life in such a way that you are not giving your immune system a chance and are therefore a sitting duck for any passing bug?

Positive and Negative Aspects of the Environment

We are used to being told that environmental factors are bad for us and I am about to argue that we need to be even more aware of how we can be affected by them. A greater recognition of the fact that our environment can affect us also raises the possibility that some aspects can have a very beneficial effect. If we take sunlight as a very obvious example, its effect on man can be both good and bad. A holiday in the sun can help us relax, revitalize us, and send us back to normal life in the British climate feeling a new person. But over-exposure to sun (and what constitutes 'over-exposure' varies from one person to the next) can cause sunburn, sunstroke and, according to some authorities, skin cancer. We need to be aware of the possible effects and discover our *individual* response. We also need to concentrate on the beneficial effects which can be an aid to healing and minimize the potentially damaging ones.

Radiation

Whether we like it or not, we are inevitably exposed to a multitude of energy frequencies or what I call, in a very general unscientific way, radiation. Technological progress has multiplied the problems of radiation and we are already aware that while some forms, such as X-ray, radar and ultra-violet, have their uses, over-exposure to them is not desirable. Many other forms, both those which occur naturally and those which are generated by technology, are not adequately recognized.

Electric and Electro-magnetic Fields

Take the national electrical grid system as an example. Many thousands of miles of high-voltage cable cross our homes, gardens, work and leisure areas. It is well known that high-voltage transmission lines can cause electrical break-down of the air in the immediate vicinity of the wires via a process known as 'corona'. This is not considered particularly serious, though it is noisy and produces ozone, a highly reactive and toxic gas which, in sufficient concentration, is harmful to animals and plants.[1] More controversial are the electric and electro-magnetic fields which the wires create.[2] Since the late 1960s a great deal of research has been done, particularly as the Russians reported that workers in electrical sub-stations were suffering various ill effects, including cardio-vascular and neurological disorders, and the electrical fields were thought to be responsible. Numerous scientists claim that electric and electro-magnetic fields affect living organisms by altering behaviour, physiology, or both.

This can include the speeding up or slowing down of responses, the development of tumours, or stunted growth. The research related to a projected submarine communications system in the United States called Project Sanguine is particularly interesting and ominous. The operating characteristics of Sanguine were similar to high-voltage transmission lines, but were about one million times weaker—and were still shown to have biological effects.

The Central Electricity Generating Board claims[3] that we have nothing to worry about. Apparently the Russians now say that they overstated the dangers and it is claimed that much of the research both on humans and animals which gave rise to concern had been deficient in some respect of scientific procedure. The general conclusions to be drawn from the evidence are, according to the Central Electricity Generating Board, reassuring, notwithstanding the odd suggestion that various health effects may occur. These suggestions include a possible connection between electric or electro-magnetic fields and congenital deformity, childhood cancer, infant death and suicide!

Other scientists, notably Marino and Becker come up with very different conclusions from the same evidence.[4] Admittedly, much of the really alarming research, whereby exposure results in death or development of tumours in animals, involves electric fields much higher that those to which we are subjected by high-voltage transmission lines. The experts cannot agree whether long-term exposure to relatively low level fields might be potentially as damaging as short-term exposure to high-level fields. In the absence of scientific concensus it would at least seem sensible to err on the side of caution when planning new lines.

We all take electrical appliances for granted and it has been rightly pointed out that we accept many risks in our daily lives in order to enjoy the advantages that advancing technology has bestowed. The trouble is that we do not always realize the possible extent of the risks we run. I have mentioned the controversy about high-voltage transmission lines as much as anything else to show that even with something as well-established as electricity we do not know all the answers, and the experts are very far from unanimous.

There are numerous other side effects of domestic technical developments which are receiving insufficient recognition. Microwave ovens[5], for example, can lead to mutations at a congenital level and can kill directly through organic damage if the shielding mechanisms are inadequate. Even television is potentially dangerous, especially a coloured set, if someone is exposed to it for too long, as one of the rays is horribly similar to X-ray which is already known to be damaging in large quantities. Less well known are the effects of inaudible vibration above and below the sonic range in some types of machinery. I was present when an engineer was rescued in the nick of time from his control room. He was rushed to hospital and it was found that the muscles in his chest had been beaten up so that they no longer worked properly and he could hardly breathe. This was finally thought to be the result of the vibrations from the experimental jet engine they were using. In this case, it was a combination of circumstances that prompted the damage. The rest of us on deck were not affected but the vibrations in the enclosed engine-room were nearly disastrous.

Countering Adverse Radiation

My children would revolt if I banned television and I am not suggesting that we abandon technology. It must make sense, however, to be aware of the potential dangers and take precautions to shield ourselves from them. As a non-scientist I am aware of some of, if not all, the dangers. Though I have no scientific rationale I have found that I can frequently offset troublesome emanations by placing patterns or strips of metal in the path of the energy, but this whole field merits far more research.

The Case for Empirical Assessment of Radiation

We do not understand the mechanism by which radiation affects us. This is still the case with electric and electro-magnetic fields as whatever molecular mechanisms may ultimately be uncovered, it is apparent that the observed effects are not energetically driven by the applied field. In other words, the fields affect us in a roundabout way which nobody quite understands. Marino and Becker suggest that the role of the field is to perturb or trigger the biological field, thereby causing it to change. Others think that the effects are brought about by ionization, one of the effects of the break-down of the air. Whatever the mechanism involved, the results are observable and they are not all bad. Some of the research has opened up the possibility that carefully controlled exposure may produce beneficial effects. Marino and Becker quote experiments by Bassett[4], for example, who found that extremely low-frequency fields increased the rate of fracture-healing in dogs and they conclude that human exposure to such fields under proper medical supervision, may be of considerable benefit to mankind.

The lack of comprehensive understanding of even electricity encourages me to think that I may not be immediately laughed down if I put forward the hypothesis that other forms of radiation affect us for good or ill. The evidence for electrical fields is circumstantial in that we do not understand the mechanism, though at least we can measure the postulated agent. I maintain (and once again I am not alone) that other radiation affects us and can circumstantially be shown to do so, though the proof of the theory is made extremely difficult by the fact that we cannot scientifically measure the radiation supposedly involved.

Places that Make Us Comfortable or Otherwise and Earth Radiation
We all know places that make us feel relaxed, happy and secure—or
the reverse. This can be partly because the place is familiar, or because
we are surrounded by people we like. It can be partly explained by
individual tastes. Some like the bustle of cities and feel lonely in the
country. Others feel at home near mountains, or the seashore or the
desert. But there is more to it than familiarity or personal taste. Some
places can make us feel particularly good or very uneasy for no
obvious reasons. In many cases, I would suggest that this is a response
to radiation from the earth.

We know that energy reaches us not only from the sun but from an
infinite number of sources, including such strange entities as quasars.
The earth itself radiates energy and it does so more strongly in certain
areas. Earth radiation can be either beneficial or detrimental to life and
some people are particularly sensitive to it. Animals and plant life are
of course also affected. Watch any group of animals and you will see
that they habitually pick the same path from one end of the field to
another, though it is frequently not the most direct or sheltered route.
Many farmers and keepers of livestock will tell you that if animals are
allowed a wide range of territory they all avoid certain areas and
congregate in others for no apparent reasons such as shelter or better
grazing.

Ley Lines and Earth Radiations
Earth energies can either well straight up out of the ground and affect
the area surrounding the spot where they surface or they can flow like
rivers, criss-crossing each other at intervals[6]. Nowadays we tend to
call these streams of energy 'ley lines', but their existence has been
known of for thousands of years. The Chinese called them 'dragon
lines' and would never consider putting up any building for human
habitation without first consulting those who were skilled in assessing
the power for good or ill of the site. Even recently, a Chinese versed in
the old knowledge told me that Western man must be considered mad
to build wherever there was a space without any regard to the possible
harm that could emanate from the spot.

As usual, the Chinese are not alone and evidence of this knowledge
is found in every culture throughout the world. Ancient temples,
shrines (later to be followed by churches) oracles, places of healing and
teaching, as well as dwelling places for people and animals were built
where strongly beneficial streams of energy crossed each other. As so
often in Europe, the vestiges of the old tradition lived on in an outdated
official title long after the knowledge had been corrupted or lost.
Geomancy (the sacred knowledge of the layout of the landscape) was
the old art and every court had its geomancer. The Court geomancer
remained an official post long after geomancy had deteriorated into

garbled hocus-pocus, defined in many an encyclopaedia as divination or even sorcery.

You may ask why ley lines are brought into a book about healing. This to me is like asking what part hygiene and sanitary housing have to play in medicine. The radiation from beneficial (so-called 'white') ley lines can give a pronounced boost to those who live within their influence. Detrimental ('black') lines can be a very strong factor in encouraging discord and illness, ranging from emotional disorder to pathological disease although probably only the latter would be recorded.

Some people are sensitive enough to feel accurately where ley lines run, but otherwise they can be traced by dowsing.[7] A group of dowsers decided to conduct some research with the help of doctors into the reality of the adverse effects of black ley lines. They wanted a contained area which would also have medical records stretching back as far as possible. They therefore chose a small British island where there had always been the tradition of so-called 'cancer houses' associated not necessarily with cancer but with severe illness. The dowsers traced a number of ley lines, including some strong black ones, and submitted their findings to those who had access to the medical records. Every house under which the black lines ran had a history of chronic illness and an unusually large number of cancer victims among its residents as far back as records could be studied.

Faced with this potential danger, I pay a great deal of attention to ley lines. A doctor treating someone with bronchitis would probably be concerned if the patient lived in a damp room and would recommend him to remedy the damp or move if at all possible. In the same way, I would find out if any adverse lines run underneath the patient's house or place of work and would offer to correct the quality of energy flow. It would seem that ley lines are subject to physical laws as it is possible to turn a black line white by a number of methods. White lines can be turned black be mining or other geological disturbance.

While I and others like me are employed to correct energy patterns at an individual level, this activity is on a very small scale and there is an enormous national and even international need to research the problem, particularly in view of the terrible disruptive effects of the major disturbances we have inflicted on the earth in the last few centuries. Think of the effects of building our enormous hospitals, schools and churches on powerfully negative sites. In the same way that many people live in a damp house with no ill effects, some will be unaffected by black lines, but this is no reason to ignore the problem, imperilling those who are susceptible.

Colour, Shape, Sound and Movement
Part of the power of particular places may be because, subjectively, we

like or dislike them. They put us in a particular mood. Mood or state of mind has been shown in the biofeedback experiments to have physiological effects. Mood can, in turn, be affected by a number of things from medical or hallucinatory drugs (be they stimulating or relaxing) to places, people, colour, form, sound and a multitude of other stimuli.

I claim that places have a force of their own, independent of the subjective likes or dislikes of the individual, and the same appears to be true of colour, shape, sound and form. In the 1930s, Ghadiali propounded the theory that colours represent chemical potencies in higher octaves of vibration, and that every organ and system can be stimulated or inhibited by the correct application of a specific colour. Undoubtedly, certain colours can stimulate or sedate an individual and many such as Steiner have developed this recognition to a very effective science. Theo Gimbel[8] is one of those who is currently applying the knowledge that both the colour and the shape of the rooms in which we live can affect us. He found that by rounding all the corners in a room he could bring enormous relief to people suffering from certain emotional or psychological disturbances. Those who design homes and offices have no idea of the powerful effect of their creations! The power of architectural design was known in the past and is gradually gaining recognition once more. At a sensational level, the shape of the pyramid of Cheops has proved to have extraordinary power. A small but exact replica can reproduce this, as if you place a blunt razor blade in it overnight, it will be sharp and clean in the morning.[9]

The pyramids appear to have a certain power which tentatively could be attributed to shape. It has been established that in certain points in the pyramid, milk and meat will remain fresh for years. Whatever the expalantion, the pyramids present problems to the scientists. In 1968, Einshams University in Cairo set up a very expensive project to excavate the pyramid of Chephren at Giza to try and find secret chambers. Computers and space age electronic equipment ran for 24 hours a day for over a year recording on magnetic tape the rays reaching the interior of the pyramid. The recordings were totaly inconsistent and from the outraged scientists' point of view, gibberish. In a letter to *The Times* of 14 July 1969, Dr Amir Golid, the scientist in charge, said the research had reached an impasse and stated that 'there is some force that defies the laws of science at work in the pyramid'.

It is thought that the power of architectural form was also known in Europe. Louis Charpentier[10] is one of those who consider that some of the cathedrals (Charpentier is particularly interested in Chartres) express esoteric knowledge and that the proportions can have very strong effects on man.

Others have found that music too can be very powerful. Music can be soothing and stimulating by turns, but certain notes and harmonies can have specific effects. Some notes, for example, can keep you awake to the point of nervous collapse. Most people have heard that certain notes can shatter a glass. Specific notes can therefore be used to produce both emotional and physiological results and this is well known in the East where, even at its simplest, each chakra is considered to 'resonate' at a certain note. I am told that this knowledge of the power of sound was still known in the Middle Ages and was used with an effect that even we can dimly appreciate in the composition of Gregorian chant, aimed to stimulate the mystic and spiritual centres of man.

Dancing or exercise in various forms can help to balance the flow of energy through the body. Some disciplines (Eastern again) have developed a science of posture and movement where each skilled and precise stance or movement has a particular physical or non-physical purpose for the practitioner. Many of these disciplines are now available in the West. Yoga, the martial arts and many of their derivatives including T'ai Chi, if properly taught, can be seen to be of enormous mental and physical benefit.

Our culture partially recognizes the effect that the loving and careful practice of an art or a skill can have, but we have no real inkling of the full importance of the complexities. Thus Music and Movement is taught as a subject in schools, and Occupational Therapy is provided in the medical field, but we still have a great deal to learn.

Nutrition[11]

In a physical sense, we are what we eat. Nutritionists of various convictions tell us that certain foods are carcinogens and they are probably right. Most people have heard that refined sugar and flour are thought to be extremely harmful in large quantities. The pesticides used on our crops can end up in your digestive systems, and many of the hormonizers, additives and chemical dyes can be damaging. It is not only the materials but the manufacturing process which can result in toxic effects. Technological progress is going so fast that monitoring standards are not keeping pace, and in many cases commercial interests are unfortunately at odds with consumer safety. Nonetheless, large numbers of people will happily survive on a supposedly unhealthy diet. Others can eat most things with impunity but will be found to be allergic to something normally considered innocuous such as wheat. While we can generalize by saying that numerous foods are potential trouble-makers, we also have to realize that one man's meat is undoubtedly another man's poison.

We do not pay nearly enough attention either to what we eat or to the many vital ingredients such as minerals which we fail to eat. The subject demands a great deal of attention and, unfortunately, I cannot do justice to it here. Nutritional good sense can be taught in general terms but, as in everything else, it is the individual reaction that matters most. A competent healer/dowser has an advantage here as he or she can immediately detect the foods to which the patient is allergic, without having to wait for the results of the conventional tests which can take several months to complete. It is worth remembering that psychological as well as physical discomfort and illness can result from eating the wrong things. To quote an extreme, it was discovered some years ago that agene, a product that was once used to bleach flour, could send laboratory research animals mad if fed to them in large quantities. It is always worth checking for dietary allergies in all disease, including non-physical disturbance, as once the allergy-producing factor has been isolated it is so easy to start the reverse process, and it can be very encouraging for someone suffering uncharacteristic depression to discover that the cause, or one of the causes, is a straightforward dietary one.

Those who find nutrition within their dowsing range will find it very useful in relation to their own health, if embarassing on occasion to their hosts. I well remember one American lady who had attended a conference of the British Society of Dowsers. She and her husband stayed on after the conference and dined with the remaining members of the group at their hotel. She was allergic to shellfish. The menu included fish with some seemingly innocuous white wine sauce. She dowsed her plateful nevertheless, and reported that her sauce contained shellfish. The waiter was summoned and challenged. He replied soothingly and not a little patronizingly. The other guests gazed around the room in the manner of embarassed Englishmen, but she stuck to her guns, and the waiter retired to confer with the chef, only to return full of apologies. Madam was quite right. The sauce on the menu had run out and the chef had made a supplementary one, this time adding shellfish. We returned to our fish, our American friend had steak and saved herself two days' food poisoning.

Bibliography

1. Marino, Andrew and Becker, Robert. 'Hazard at a Distance—Effects of Exposure to the Electric and Magnetic Fields of High Voltage Transmission Lines'. *Medical Research Engineering* Vol. 12, No. 5.
2. Battocletti, Joseph H. *Electromagnetism, Man and the Environment*. Elek Scientific Books, 1976.
3. Male, J. C. and Norris, W. T. Central Electricity Research Laboratories. Laboratory Note No. RD/L/N2/80, December 1980.
4. Marino, Andrew A. and Becker, Robert. 'Biological Effects of

Extremely Low Frequency Electric and Magnetic Fields—A Review'. *Physiological Chemistry and Physics* Vol. 9, No. 2, 1977.

5. Hildyard, N. 'Overexposed'. *The New Ecologist* Vol. 9, No. 1, Jan/Feb 1979.

6. Devereux, Paul and Thomson, Ian. *The Ley Hunter's Companion.* Thames and Hudson, 1980.

7. Graves, Tom. *Dowsing: Techniques and Applications.* Turnstone Press, 1976.

8. Gimbel, Theo. *Healing Through Colour.* C. W. Daniel, 1980.

9. Watson, Lyall. *Supernature.* Coronet, 1974.

10. Charpentier, Louis. *The Mysteries of Chartres Cathedral.* Research Into Lost Knowledge Organization, 1972 (available from Thorsons).

11. This is a vast subject, but my wife Patricia, who is a much greater expert than myself, suggests that the following could form an introduction:

Lappe, Frances Moore. *Diet for a Small Planet.* Ballantine Books, 1976.

Rodale, J. I. and staff. *Complete Book of Food and Nutrition.* Rodale Books. 1961.

Davis, Adelle. *Let's Get Well.* Allen and Unwin, 1979.

Westberg, Marita. *Eat Well, Live Longer.* Quartet Books, 1979.

12. Healing Today

A recent survey of 'complementary medicine'[1] (as the authors designate it) reckons that there are over 20,000 healers practising in the UK. Given such a choice and given also the multitude of beliefs held and methods used, it is hardly surprising that anyone seeking help should feel a little bewildered. A dowser competent in this area can tell an individual which therapies are likely to be most helpful to him or her, but it is impossible to give any general guidelines. The only answer is to do a little personal research and find out which therapies and which individuals you find helpful. For the individual is very important; you may go to a very competent and successful healer with no results, and yet respond to another. Even Harry Edwards, whom I would regard as the most outstanding healer of his day, would on occasion recognize that he was not the best person to give help, and that a particular patient would respond better to healing through another person or group, and he would refer the patient accordingly. It would seem that, in some instances, patient and healer cannot for some reason 'tune in' properly. We can observe a similar occurrence with hi-fi equipment; you can have an excellent amplifier, superb turntable and all the rest, but if the mix is wrong, you will not get good musical reproduction.

Standards
Given the diversity of healers and this dependence on the individual reaction, it is very difficult to asses who is a 'good' healer and who is a 'bad' one. This leaves the field open to delusion and even abuse. People are particularly vulnerable when they are ill, and in their desire to get well, can become very gullible. There are and always have been those who will cash in on this human weakness. There is no easy answer to this, and to say that there are, always have been and probably always will be charlatans in the healing field as in every other field is not a good reason for ignoring the field itself. The difficulty is in distinguishing the good from the bad, the self-deluded and incompetent from the

genuinely effective. In fields such as medicine and the law, we have on the whole managed to minimize abuses by setting up high standards of examination and strict codes with an established body to monitor conduct and complaints. It would make life very much easier if we could do the same in the healing field.

There is the obvious need for society to be protected from the antics of dangerous individuals, but there is also the need for the individual to be protected from domination by any particular group, be it political, commercial, religious or anything else. We have to keep the balance always in view so that, at one extreme, abuses are minimized and at the other that a monopoly does not impede the growth of new ideas. Standards and codes are extremely useful, but it is vital to recognize that they must change from time to time in the light of changing circumstances or new discoveries.

We are extremely fortunate in Britain in that medical codes now leave the door open for doctors to liaise with healers, but we are still left with the problem of assessing healers. It would be convenient if we had some measurable standard by which to judge them. At this point I think it is important to distinguish between the many therapies that are used as adjuncts to healing, and the simple acts of laying on hands and absent healing. It would be possible and perhaps desirable to set up standards of practice for some therapies (such as massage), though we have to be on the alert to incorporate improvements. Until we can establish a relevant yardstick it would be extremely difficult, and not necessarily desirable, to set up standards for simple healing. While it is undoubtedly useful for healers to have a basic knowlege of anatomy, it is not by any means essential, and to insist upon learnt knowledge when assessing an intuitive gift is not necessarily relevant or satisfactory. If academic examinations became a prerequisite for healers, a great deal of valuable assistance would be outlawed. (Incidentally, I have heard doubts expressed, even in medical circles, about the increasing dependence on academic qualifications. The medical schools are naturally tempted to choose the most academically brilliant students, who qualify with distinction, but unless they have that 'extra something' which you might call a genuine vocation, they do not necessarily make good doctors.)

Some criteria other than academic also cause me concern. Healing works regardless of the belief system of practitioner or patient, and any attempt to set up codes of practice might bring with it a tendency to encourage one set of beliefs rather than another, and to establish a new closed shop.

The National Federation of Spiritual Healers continually wrestles with the problem of standards, but so far has found it impossible to do anything but establish very basic criteria for membership, involving the subjective testimony of a small number of supposedly successful patients. It would be much more satisfactory if the medical profession could be persuaded to extend their current tolerance to active co-operation in arranging more 'before and after studies' of patients. Perhaps biofeedback tests could be helpful in assessing whether a healer is in fact capable of tuning in to the brain wave pattern which seems to be associated with healing and called by Cade 'state five'. As long as there are no established standards, it is unfortunately up to individuals to keep their critical faculties intact and evaluate whether they or others they know have been helped or not.

The Law

We are extremely fortunate in Britain in that the law allows practitioners of 'alternative' medicine considerable freedom. There are laws quite rightly preventing healers from poaching on the preserves of the medical profession in certain areas as, for example, in the prescription of drugs, where expert knowledge is essential. By and large, however, healers are allowed to operate as they wish, and it is up to individual doctors to liaise with them if they wish to. We are seeing a gradual change of attitude, and I devoutly hope that the co-operation and trust between healers and doctors will grow.

The legal situation is very different in other countries. At one extreme, Brazil accepts healing as a useful branch of medicine and healers are an integrated part of many hospitals. A recent government-appointed commission[2] in Holland recommends that the Dutch Government should go the same way so that healing would be available within the official health service and insurance schemes. Germany gives healers the oportunity to join the ranks of the establishment by offering a lay qualification. The academic standard is quite high, I am told, so that a number of effective healers (who are not necessarily great brains) are excluded. The other European countries are, at least officially, less in sympathy with healing and there is always the worry that EEC attempts to standardize the position will result in the triumph of a less tolerant attitude. Questions recently raised at the European Parliament about tightening up the law on various aspects of alternative medicine received an evasive answer, however, and it would seem that, at least for the moment, the legislators have no wish to stir up a hornet's nest. Meanwhile, we must hope that doctors and healers will work together more closely in Britain and that further research will help to establish a more comprehensive rationale with which to combat any intolerant legislation.

Healing appears to be growing and attracting more and more interest in the USA, despite the law, which in certain States is so strict that it is illegal for a lay healer even to touch his patient. Despite official restrictions on practice, theory is receiving greater attention than it is in Europe, and American research seems likely to shed increasing light on healing and on all other branches of the supposedly paranormal.

Payment

Wherever healers may choose to practise they are usually confronted with the question of whether they should charge for their services or not. Obviously there have been (and probably always will be) some who cash in on the vulnerability of people desperate to get well. Leaving aside the deliberate frauds, there are many who feel that it is wrong to charge money for exercising a God-given gift. Yet, by this argument, all our gifts are God-given and a musician, an artist, or a businessman using his numerate abilty, all patently have to earn their living by using their respective talents. The difficulty lies in the absence of any observable standards of healing. A musician or an artist can be judged on aesthetic or technical grounds and will only earn a living if he satisfies the criteria of his public. I feel that anyone believing that he or she is a healer should be careful about charging anyone to begin with. Only if he satisfies himself (and his patients!) that he really can help others, should he consider charging. I practised healing in my spare time for nearly twenty years and never charged during that time. But then I did not need to: I had my army pay, and for most of that time I was a bachelor. By the time I left the army I had my wife, Patricia, to consider. She encouraged me in my determination to continue with healing and to this end we bought our little house in Fife. It did not seem sensible to me to give up all other forms of support, so to begin with healing remained a spare-time activity; and to feed us and the first of our three sons who appeared in 1959 I had my small army pension and a job as a pigman on a nearby large farm. More and more people began to come for healing; however, the numbers became more than I could cope with in my spare time. It was at this point that we decided that I should devote all my time to healing and that in this case I should have to charge my patients. I have done so ever since and feel that, provided a healer has honestly satisfied himself (or herself) that he really can help others, then it is fair to earn a living from his endeavours.

The Way Ahead

Our world is changing fast and it is to be hoped that governments and individuals will continue honestly to try and assess the work of various intuitive forms of knowledge and abilities which we have ignored for too long. The development of increasingly sophisticated scientific instruments is showing that many aspects can already be seen as natural rather than supernatural. As Koestler says, '. . . the odour of the alchemist's kitchen is replaced by the smell of quark in the laboratory'.[3] There is increasing interest in the supposedly paranormal and this goes both for observed phenomena such as healing and for the age-old contention of the world religions that we can experience a benevolent, non-physical power which appears to be partly or wholly beyond and far greater than the individual self.

Bibliography
1. Fulder. Stephen and Monro, Robin. *The Status of Complementary Medicine in the United Kingdom.* Threshold Foundation, 1981.
2. 'Alternative Medicine in the Netherlands'. Summary of the Report of the Commission for Alternative Systems of Medicine. The Hague, 1981.
3. Koestler, Arthur. *The Roots of Coincidence.* Pan Books, 1976.

13. Conclusion: The Soul

Those who turned to this book in the expectation of finding a cut-and-dried explanation for the existence of some healing capacity in man are bound to be disappointed. As a sop to the rational man who finds talk of extended awareness (not to mention discarnate existence) both distasteful and unsettling, may I stress yet again that healing *works*, regardless of belief and that at least some aspects of this phenomenon are coming within the grasp of science.

Biofeedback, the work with trypsin and probably Kirlian photography show that purported healing has measurable correlates. This, however, is not and never will be the whole story. Healing is only one aspect of human potential which Western man, for reasons of mental conditioning, is reluctant to look at. He is like one of the inhabitants of Plato's cave, an allegory in *The Republic* which is perhaps worth quoting[1], even for the many who know it already.

'Let me show in allegory how far our nature is enlightened or unenlightened. Imagine human beings living in an underground cave, which has a mouth open toward the light and reaching all along the cave. Here they have been from childhood. They have their legs and necks chained so that they cannot move and can only see the wall of the cave before them, being prevented by the chains from turning their heads. Above and behind them at a distance the fire of the sun is blazing and between the sun and the prisoners there is a raised way and a low wall built along the way. And do you see men passing along the way carrying all sorts of vessels and statues and figures of animals made of wood and stone and various materials which appear as shadows on the wall of the cave facing the prisoners? Some of them are talking, others silent.'

'You have shown me a strange image and they are strange prisoners', Glaucon replies.

'Like ourselves, and they see only their own shadows, or the shadows which the sun throws on the opposite wall of the cave, of the men and the objects which are being carried. If they were able to converse with one another, would they not suppose that they were seeing as realities what was before them? And suppose further that the prison had an echo which

came from the other side. Would they not be sure to fancy when one of
the passers-by spoke that the voice which they heard came from the
passing shadow? To them the truth would be literally but the shadows of
images.

'At first, when any one of the prisoners is liberated and compelled
suddenly to stand up and turn around and walk and look towards the
light he will suffer sharp pain and he will be unable to see the reality of
which in his former state he had seen the shadow. Conceive of someone
saying to him that what he saw before was an illusion. Would he not be
perplexed? Would he not fancy that the shadows which he formerly saw
are truer than the objects which are now shown to him? If he is compelled
to look straight at the light, will he not have a pain in his eyes which will
make him turn away? He will take refuge in the shadows which he can see
and which he will conceive to be in reality clearer than the things which
are now being shown to him?

'He will require to grow accustomed to the sight of the upper world.
Last of all, he will be able to see the sun. He will then proceed to argue that
the sun is he who gives the seasons and the years and is the guardian of all
that is in the visible world, and in a certain way the cause of all things
which he and his fellows have been accustomed to behold.

'When he remembered his old habitation and the wisdom of the cave
and his fellow prisoners, do you suppose that he would congratulate
himself on the change and pity them? Imagine once more such an
individual coming suddenly out of the sun to be replaced in his old
situation. Would he not be certain to have his eyes full of darkness?

'If there were contests and he had to compete in measuring the shadows
with the prisoners who had never moved out of the cave, while his sight
was still weak, would he not seem ridiculous? They would say of him,
"Up he went and down he came without his eyes", and that it would be
better not even to think of ascending. If anyone tried to loose another and
lead him up to the light, let them only catch the offender and they would
put him to death.'

I hope I am not labouring the point if I elaborate Plato's analogy for
my own puposes. Science and technology have already placed man, at
least intellectually, a little closer to the entrance of the cave, in a new
environment which is pure energy moving in swift and ever-changing
patterns of frequency. His concepts of his world built on the experience
of a limited use of five senses is no longer adequate and, in many cases,
no longer valid.

Let us assume that by 'extending our awareness' we are like an
inhabitant of the cave who comes back and demonstrates that he can
play football or stand on his head. His fellows will find this 'unnatural'.
I would maintain that much that is currently considered 'unnatural', be
it healing, clairvoyance, telepathy, levitation, mediumship, the ability
such as that of Yuri Geller to move or affect objects without touching
them, or any of the phenomena described consistently throughout the
millenia are similarly not 'unnatural', they are simply latent
capabilities awaiting rediscovery.

Those who return to the cave and talk about or demonstrate their new-found discoveries may well call them different things. The amount they have learnt will vary, and the use they make of their discoveries is equally a matter of choice. Thus we have arguments over terminology, though the phenomena themselves are unchanging. 'Psychic' and 'medium' are now almost dirty words to some people, but synonyms are becoming acceptable. 'Parapsychology' is almost respectable. Shafica Karagulla[2] came to the conclusion after much research that many people demonstrate 'higher sense perception', in which she includes clairvoyant diagnosis, the ability to see and affect energy fields and telepathic assistance. Her research is fascinating and we can, I hope, look forward to additional enlightenment from the Higher Sense Perception Research Foundation in Beverley Hills. Karagulla differentiates between the ways people use their abilities, but the abilities themselves, whether they be called 'higher sense perception', 'extra sensory perception', 'psychic' or anything else remain identical. As already mentioned, I myself prefer the term 'extended sensory perception'.

Some may return to the cave having mastered only a little of a skill and with a very poor understanding of what they have seen. They can do party tricks which are of no particular use to anyone except at a sensational level of entertainment. Their explanations can be misleading. Some may have attained a greater understanding but few if any will comprehend the full complexity of the outside world they have visited. They cannot become versed in physics, biology, biochemistry and all the other spheres of knowledge let alone in the arts all at once. At the moment, we have good reason to mistrust those who claim to have a monopoly of the truth, and to be particularly suspicious of those who have not visited the outside world or at least paid only fleeting visits and yet set up dogmatic institutions claiming to be the only authority on the subject. No amount of teaching by those who have ventured out of the cave, no matter how enlightened, coherent and undogmatic they may be, can take the place of personal experience.

Plato assumed that our allegorical cave dweller comes straight out of the gloom into brilliant, blinding sunlight. He assumes that he will quickly realize that the sun is '. . . in a certain way the cause of all things which he and his fellows have been accustomed to behold'. The idea of power, of energy preceding and permeating all life in our universe is not new. Light has always been the symbol of greater understanding, of 'enlightenment'. There are many who observe the power of the sun without experiencing a qualitative change in their understanding or consciousness. Many others, however, try to describe in their different ways their individual experience of being part of a greater, enlightened cosmic consciousness. Their experiences are variously described as religious, transcendental and spiritual. William James[3] and more recently Alister Hardy[4] have studied these 'subjective' experiences with considerable erudition. They analyze profound similarities in the types of experience and James concludes that' . . . so long as we deal with the cosmic and general, we deal only with the symbols of reality, but as soon as we deal with private and personal phenomena as such we deal with realities in the completest sense of the term'. This is to insist that in such studies there is no possibility of eliminating a subjective component. Should it be thought that a subjective component invalidates the studies, it should be remembered that even the physicists now conclude that no experiment in the subatomic field can be totally objective as the observer is always automatically involved in an essential way.

Many others describe experiences similar to the visionaries and the yogis through the use of drugs. There is often the fear of the *mysterium tremens* (the blinding sunlight?) and the feeling of losing the 'self' and entering a transcendental world. With these qualitative changes of consciousness comes an ethical conception, or perhaps a 'spiritual' perception which goes beyond ethics. Koestler[5] may say a little drily that ' . . . the need for self-transcendence through some form of "peak experience" . . . is inherent in man's condition . . .' and that ' . . . transcendental beliefs are derived from certain ever-recurrent archetypal patterns which evoke instant emotive responses . . .', but he is observing both a need and a reality. The result is the ever-recurring theme that man aspires to union with a spiritual force and that only when he recognizes this can he live to the full. Aldous Huxley[6] put it another way:

> . . . the quietists may not practise contemplation in its fullness, but if they practise it at all, they may bring back enlightened reports of another, a transcendent country of the mind; and if they practise it in the height, they will become conduits through which some beneficent influence can flow out of that other country into a world of darkened selves, chronically dying for lack of it.

Here we have the view that some 'beneficent influence' can flow through man to his fellow humans. This 'beneficent influence' can be seen both as 'enlightenment', and also some more concrete 'stuff' with power to affect the material world. This has always been the religions' point about prayer. Frederic W. H. Myers, in a letter to a friend quoted by William James[3], is explicit.

> I am glad that you have asked me about prayer, because I have rather strong ideas on the subject. First consider the facts. There exists around us a spiritual universe and that universe is in actual relation with the material. From the spiritual universe comes the energy which maintains the material; the energy which makes the life of each individual spirit. . .

Plainly we must endeavour to draw in as much spiritual life as possible, and we must place our minds in any attitude which experience shows favourable to such indrawal. Prayer is the general name for that attitude of open and earnest expectancy. If we then ask to *whom* we pray, the answer (strangely enough) must be that that does not much matter. The prayer is not indeed a purely subjective thing, it means a real increase in intensity of absorption of spiritual power or grace but we do not know enough of what takes place in the spiritual world to know how that prayer operates.

The point he makes is that in prayer (and, in my view, potentially in any of the other means of extending awareness) spiritual energy, which otherwise would slumber, does become active and spiritual work of some kind is effected in the physical world.

It is important that in Myer's words the spiritual world 'is in actual relation to the material' and in some aspects presumably permeates physical forces. In other words, we can observe and measure these physical forces without considering the spiritual power which permeates them. In relation to healing, some facets may be scientifically measurable, but in my view are dependent upon the spiritual order whether this is recognized or not. If I may hark back once more to Plato's troglodytes, it is quite possible that an individual could come out of the cave on a day when the sun was hidden behind the clouds. He could go back and recount what he had seen and show what he had learnt, but he would not realize that there was any 'guardian of all that is in the visible world' or 'a cause of all things which he and his fellows have been accustomed to behold'.

It is important to distinguish between the sun's energy and power and its blinding light. Power is of itself neutral, it *is*. We can harness it, whatever classification of energy it may be, to heal or harm. It is our motivation and state of understanding or enlightenment which determine the use to which we put it. We may even put it to beneficial use with little or no real spiritual aspiration. The Master, Jesus, pointed out the distinction between power and spiritual enlightenment when he talked of 'false Christs'. Such men would be able to harness power, to perform 'miracles'. From the point of view of those who received help and healing this would be a very good thing, but from the point of view of pointing out man's real goal authoritatively and helping him to spiritual advancement, their teaching would be misleading. The Tibetans recognize a similar distinction. They consider the attainment of 'psychic' power as well within the capacity of man and extremely beneficial if used properly. They stress that such attainment is not an end in itself as it should lead to spiritual growth. If it does become an end in itself then it can constitute a distraction from the true path.

Much that man is currently studying leads to some inkling of a spiritual world. Scientists in various fields and psychologists frequently find their work leading them into unexpected dimensions. The Wrekin Trust, (see page 124) now runs an annual conference entitled 'Mystics and Scientists', two groups who for years have been thought totally opposed and now find themselves grappling with similar experiences. The 1982 conference included the eminent neurophysiologist and Nobel prizewinner Sir John Eccles F.R.S., who argues not only that mind has an existence independent of the brain but also that human evolution is not a series of fortuitous accidents and that we are creatures with some supernatural meaning.[7] Dr Lawrence Le Shan[8] is another who points out the underlying similarities of understanding between widely divergent disciplines in his book *Clairvoyant Reality*.

The spiritual renaissance, as we could call it, gains additional momentum from the re-emergence not only of religious practices but of physical disciplines originating in the East. Many people, perturbed by the physiological effects of sedentary urban life take up 'exercise classes'. The physiological effects of yoga, T'ai Chi and a multitide of other disciplines are undoubtedly extremely helpful, but once again the student, whether he intended it or not, is lead towards a recognition of spiritual reality. Man is body, mind and spirit and he can operate in wholeness, in an integration of all his potential. This way lies the only fully effective path to freedom from 'dis-ease'. You may regard soul and spirit as aspects of mind or as separate entities in themselves. Some schools of thought consider soul and spirit as the same thing, others distinguish between them and create further sub-divisions. The distinctions do not matter very much at this point. The important thing is to recognize the broad dimensions of man and the interplay between them. By changing one we may change another. The work with biofeedback instruments is only one of the many areas of research which are showing the physiological reality of the effect of mind. The very acceptance of psychiatry, psychology and psychotherapy shows that orthodox medicine is already at least recognizing that mechanical failure in the body cannot be totally divorced from emotional and mental well-being. There are many others who claim that the search for true health, be it of individuals or of society, is tied up with the search for the soul.

We desperately need all the medical skills available today and healing should not be seen as a substitute. It is essentially complementary. While some research (with, I hope, very much more to follow) corroborates that healing which recognizes mind and spirit can help at a physiological level, it is perhaps the concept of wholeness that is most important. We lost sight of wholeness many centuries ago when religion and medicine separated. The entire well-being of man used to be embraced within the temple, but we lost this integration when certain types of knowledge came to be seen as secular and scientific and were approached separately. It would seem that untiring research in all aspects of knowledge is leading towards a dawning recognition that the old concepts of wholeness are a reality.

I believe that we can approach wholeness from any angle. The vicious circle of illness, unhappiness, strain, dissatisfaction, unrest and all the malaise of modern man can be broken at innumerable points and for this we need all the specialist skills that are available. Whilst in many cases the easiest place to start is the relief of physical symptoms, we must keep in sight the vision of man in his entirety. I would question his order of priorities, but Plato[1] expressed the necessity of a co-ordinated approach towards the whole person when he said:

> The cure of the part should not be attempted without treatment of the whole. No attempt should be made to cure the body without the soul, and, if the head and body are to be healthy, you must begin by curing the mind. That is the first thing. Let no-one persuade you to cure the body until he has first given you his soul to be cured. For this is the great error of our day in the treatment of the human body, that physicians first separate the soul from the body.

Bibliography

1. Plato. *The Republic*. Pan Books, 1981.
2. Karagulla, Shafica. *Breakthrough to Creativity*. De Vorss, 1967.
3. James, William. *The Varieties of Religious Experience*. The Gifford Lectures, delivered at Edinburgh 1901-2. First issued in the Fontana Library, 1960.
4. Hardy, Sir Alister. *The Spiritual Nature of Man*. Oxford University Press, 1979.
5. Koestler, Arthur. *The Ghost in the Machine*. Hutchinson, 1976.
6. Huxley, Aldous. *The Doors of Perception*. Panther, 1977.
7. Eccles, Sir John Carew. *'The Human Mystery'*. Gifford Lectures, 1977-78. Springer International, 1979.
8. Le Shan, Dr Lawrence. *Clairvoyant Reality*. Turnstone Press, 1980.

Useful Addresses

Audio Ltd.
(Designers and manufacturers of Biofeedback equipment)
26 Wendell Road
London
W12 9RT

The British Society of Dowsers
Sycamore Cottage
Tamley Lane
Hastingleigh
Ashford
Kent
TN25 5HW

College of Psychic Studies
16 Queensberry Place
London
SW7 2EB

De la Warr Laboratories (Radionics)
Raleigh Park Road
Oxford

Institute for Complementary Medicine
21 Portland Place
London
W1N 3AF

Institute for Psychobiological Research
2 Ulysses Road
London
NW6

The Medical and Scientific Network
Lake House
Ockley
Nr. Dorking
Surrey
RH5 5NS

National Federation of Spiritual Healers
Old Manor Farm Studio
Sunbury on Thames
Middx

Society for Psychical Research
1 Adam and Eve Mews
London
W8 6UG

The Westbank Healing and Teaching Centre
Strathmiglo
Fife
KY14 7QP

White Eagle Lodge
Newlands Rake
Liss
Hampshire
GU33 7HY

The Wrekin Trust
Dove House
Little Birch
Hereford HR2 8BB

Index